The Immobilized Patient

Functional Pathology and Management

TOPICS IN BONE AND MINERAL DISORDERS

Series Editor: Louis V. Avioli, M.D.
Washington University School of Medicine
St. Louis, Missouri

A Continuation Order Plan is available for this series. A continuation order will bring delivery of each new volume immediately upon publication. Volumes are billed only upon actual shipment. For further information please contact the publisher.

The Immobilized Patient

Functional Pathology and Management

Franz U. Steinberg, M.D.

Washington University School of Medicine
and The Jewish Hospital of St. Louis

PLENUM MEDICAL BOOK COMPANY
New York and London

Library of Congress Cataloging in Publication Data

Steinberg, Franz U   1913-
    The immobilized patient.

    (Topics in bone and mineral disorders)
    Includes index.
    1. Hypokinesia. 2. Hypokinesia–Physiological aspects. I. Title. II. Series. [DNLM:
1. Immobilization. WE168 s819i]
RB135.S73   616.7   79-25903
ISBN 978-1-4684-3655-6   ISBN 978-1-4684-3653-2 (eBook)
DOI 10.1007/978-1-4684-3653-2

© 1980 Plenum Publishing Corporation
Softcover reprint of the hardcover 1st edition 1980
227 West 17th Street, New York, N.Y. 10011

Plenum Medical Book Company is an imprint of Plenum Publishing Corporation

Foreword

Teach us to live that we may dread
Unnecessary time in bed
Get people up and we may save
Our patients from an early grave.

A most revealing paraphrase by Asher* of a verse by Bishop
Thomas Ken more than adequately summarizes the plight of
the immobilized patient, who often lies dormant and depressed for years on end. In this volume, Dr. Steinberg has
offered the reader a unique opportunity to share his many
years of experience in caring for the immobilized patient. His
careful attempt to explore the pathophysiologic effects of
immobilization on a number of organ systems, combined
with a host of practical aspects with regard to patient care, is
unique and refreshing. This text should command the re-
spect of any physician faced with the vicissitudes and frus-
trations of caring for the immobilized. The final chapter de-
tailing "The Psychological Aspects of Immobilization," by
Hammer and Kenan, offers the reader considerable insight
into the essentials and value of occupational and physical
therapy. It should prove most valuable to physicians as well

*Asher, R. A. J. Dangers of going to bed. *Br. Med. J.* 2:907, 1947.

as social workers, paramedical personnel, and the many physical therapists who come into daily contact with the nonambulatory patient.

L. V. Avioli

St. Louis

Preface

It may be a paradox that the importance of disability and immobilization has been enhanced by the very progress of medical science. The advances in diagnostic and therapeutic skills let many patients survive diseases and trauma which would have doomed them in decades past. The price of survival, however, may be a permanent or temporary disability which may include long periods of immobilization. The morbidity of a long-term illness or injury is often, in part, caused by the immobilization that circumstances have imposed upon the patient. It is important, therefore, to realize that immobilization carries a morbidity of its own which can be modified and ameliorated by appropriate management. The original charge to me was to prepare a text on "The Management of the Immobilized Patient." It soon became apparent that it is not possible to deal with therapy and management without discussing the pathophysiologic effects of immobilization. As a result, the scope of the book was broadened and the title was changed to *The Immobilized Patient*.

The book does not purport to cover every aspect of immobilization. I have concentrated my attention on those organ systems which are most affected and in which the effects of immobilization contribute most to the patient's morbidity. These will be the areas of greatest importance to the clinician, who carries the final responsibility for the immobilized patient's welfare.

I would like to express my appreciation to Dr. Louis V. Avioli for his valuable help and advice; to Dr. Randy L. Hammer and Miss Emily H. Kenan for writing the chapter on the psychological aspects of immobilization; to my secretary, Mrs. Mary Pelchman, for her help in preparing the manuscript through many drafts; and to my wife, Lisl R. Steinberg, for her patience and encouragement.

Franz U. Steinberg

St. Louis

Contents

CHAPTER 1

General Aspects of Immobilization

Man's body is organized for motion. The instrument of mobility, skeletal muscle, makes up 40 percent of the body mass. Its structure and metabolic capability permit an efficient and almost instantaneous shift from complete rest to a high level of activity. As a muscle becomes active, its blood flow may rise 15 to 20 times over the resting value, and the number of open capillaries may increase 50 times. The metabolic rate of the working muscle may be 50 to 100 times above that of a muscle at rest.

The working muscle needs to be supplied with nutrients and oxygen. Metabolic waste and carbon dioxide need to be removed. The burden of this task falls upon the circulation and respiration. These organ systems are well suited to adapt to the demands of increased muscular activity. During moderate exercise the cardiac output may increase threefold; the heart rate may double. The left ventricular work may rise to 3.5 times more than resting value and the oxygen uptake per minute 6 times that seen at rest. The minute volume of respiration may increase from 5 to 7 liters to more than 50 liters. In heavy exercise, the tidal volume may be as high as 50 percent of the vital capacity.[1]

The capacity of circulation and respiration to adapt to the demands of muscular activity and of stress in general falls within the general concept of "physical fitness." This potential is furthered by physical training and is sharply reduced by immobilization. Training not only strengthens muscles; it also enhances the functional capabilities of the cardiovascular and respiratory systems. Fitness cannot be maintained without the stimulus of muscular activity. During immobilization physical fitness declines rapidly. The resting heart rate is increased. The cardiac output and the left ventricular work no longer rise sufficiently during even mild activity, and the immobile upright position is poorly tolerated. This will be discussed in more detail in Chapter 2.

Immobilization slows the response of the nervous system. A patient who is confined to bed for a long period of time becomes dull and his intellectual capabilities diminish. Depending upon his premorbid personality, the patient may become depressed, anxious, lethargic, dependent, and disassociated from family and society (see Chapter 7 for details).

The ability to perform precisely coordinated movements is also adversely affected by prolonged inactivity. The pyramidal and extrapyramidal systems make it possible to gear the force of muscular contractions to the task at hand. The activation of some muscles and the inhibition of others is the key to the precise coordination of skilled motor activity. Sensory feedback from muscles, tendons, and joints allows for the instantaneous correction of errors. This remarkable coordination of muscular activity is achieved without volitional input. Our will only directs the motor system to perform a specific task, to walk through the room, to pick up a book, etc. The needed coordination that makes some muscles contract and others relax and that gauges the force of muscular contractions is an automatic function that takes place at a subcortical level. When an individual has been immobilized for some time, the nervous system loses its capacity to coordinate movements quickly and efficiently. A patient arising from bed for the first time after a long period of confinement will stagger about. His legs do not obey his commands. The muscles, of course, are weak from long disuse but the ability to perform skilled movements has also diminished; it will take several days until this function has been regained.

The gastrointestinal tract is also affected by prolonged immobilization. The appetite is diminished. This may be advantageous since the reduced energy output requires a lower caloric intake. Unfortunately, the appetite for protein-rich foods is often selectively depressed, and this adds to the considerable net protein loss engendered by long recumbency. The constipation associated with inactivity is well known and may be difficult to manage. In elderly patients with a depressed sensorium, immobilization may lead to a fecal impaction. Often this is not suspected because the patient may have frequent liquid stools around the impaction. Since constipation further contributes to the loss of appetite, and the diminished intake of food and liquids aggravates the constipation, a vicious cycle develops.

Bladder evacuation may be inhibited by bed rest; the bladder may become distended, and overflow incontinence may be the result. A man with a hypertrophy of the prostate may develop a complete retention once confined to bed. Browse has pointed out that in the recumbent position urine may stagnate in the renal pelves.[2] In the erect body position, the hilus is almost the lowest point of the renal pelvis and only a few calices are situated below the hilar level. In the recumbent position the hilus is uppermost and all calices are positioned below. Gravity cannot aid in the expulsion of urine from the renal pelvis and the urine may remain stagnant. Calculi may form because the osteoporosis of immobilization causes an excessive excretion of calcium salts which may precipitate in a concentrated urine.

Immobilization, therefore, not only weakens muscles; it reduces the plasticity of many organ systems, their ability to adjust to changing environmental circumstances and demands. The immobilized patient no longer can adequately respond to stress. His margins of safety are sharply reduced.

The risks engendered by prolonged inactivity have been known for a long time, but systematic investigations are of relatively recent vintage. The first study of this type was published by Deitrick, Whedon, and Shorr in 1948.[3] This classic study will be cited repeatedly in subsequent sections of this volume, but the most important findings will be presented in this introductory chapter. Four healthy men were placed on 6 to 8 weeks of strict bed rest. Their movements were further restricted by the application of plaster casts. Their metabolic and circulatory functions were thoroughly investigated. Nitrogen excretion began to increase on the fifth or sixth day of immobilization. The total nitrogen loss for the four subjects averaged 53.6 g. The creatine tolerance was reduced, commensurate with the degree of muscular atrophy. One subject, who had the greatest nitrogen loss, showed a significant lowering of the 17-ketosteroid excretion. The basal metabolic rate declined at an average of 6.9 percent. The changes in body weight were small; as muscle protein was lost, fat and carbohydrate storage increased. The excretion of calcium, phosphorus, sulfate, sodium and potassium increased, with total calcium loss ranging from 9 to 24 g and phosphorus excretion paralleling that of calcium. The excess sulfate excretion correlated with the loss of nitrogen since both were due to the catabolism of muscle protein. The resting heart rate rose steadily. In the later periods of immobilization the individuals had lost much of their ability to maintain an erect posture without becoming hypotensive.

The recovery was slow. Calcium, nitrogen, and phosphorus were retained to make up for the losses during immobilization, but it took more than six weeks to establish a normal equilibrium.

In 1965, N. L. Browse published a monograph, *The Physiology and Pathology of Bed Rest.*[2] This monograph explores in detail the physiologic effects of assuming a supine position in general and of prolonged bed rest in particular. The material is based on the author's own observations and on a review of the literature. The perusal of this monograph makes it clear that there is no bodily function that is not affected by prolonged bed rest.

A number of thorough investigations on the physiologic effects of immobilization have been published by the staff of the Texas Institute for Rehabilitation and Research. A summary of their findings was published in 1965.[4] The advent of space flights has evoked a great deal of interest in the problems of immobilization because the state of weightlessness produces very similar changes in body organ function. Furthermore, astronauts spend a considerable time in the cramped quarters of their space capsule and are, in fact, immobilized by their environment.

Therapeutic Implications of Bed Rest

Browse points out that up to the middle of the 19th century, sick people took to their beds only when they were so ill that they could no longer stay up, and this they did most reluctantly. In 1863, John Hilton published a book entitled *Rest and Pain: The Influence of Mechanical and Physiological Rest in the Treatment of Accidents and Surgical Diseases and the Diagnostic Value of Pain.* In this book Hilton propounded the healing powers of rest. He explained that just as a surgeon would heal a broken bone by immobilizing it, other diseased organs could be successfully treated when the body as a whole was put to rest. Therefore bed rest for the treatment of all kinds of ailments became fashionable, and, as happens so often, rest was prescribed indiscriminately without much consideration of its possible deleterious effects.

There are, of course, conditions for which bed rest is beneficial. The patient with an acute infection, such as influenza, will do best to spend a few days in bed. Often weakness will force the patient to bed as it is. An acute myocardial infarction is treated with strict bed rest, at least for the first few days. In fact, it has been shown that the work of the heart is at its lowest when the patient is in a sitting position. The recumbent position does not rest the heart. Many years ago S. Levine suggested armchair management of patients with acute myocardial infarctions.[5] Although this suggestion has not been routinely accepted by many cardiologists, the duration of bed confinement has been sharply reduced. As little as 15 or 20 years ago, a patient with a myocardial infarction was kept in bed for 3 weeks and remained in the hospital for 6 weeks. Now the average accepted period of hospitalization for uncomplicated myocardial infarctions and other cardiac disorders is 3 weeks; patients are permitted out of bed and allowed to be active after a few days. The only apparent exception is cardiomyopathy, in which prolonged rest appears to be beneficial.

Acute hepatitis is usually treated with bed rest. This form of treatment had its origin during World War II when it was shown that soldiers had a quicker recovery and fewer relapses when kept in bed. There is some doubt that this observation carries over to civilian medicine, and over the years the prescription of strict bed rest has been modified.

Some rheumatologists have recommended that patients with acute rheumatoid arthritis be treated with strict bed rest in a sanatorium fashion.[6] This has not been universally accepted, and its value has not been demonstrated.

The well-established use of bed rest in the treatment of pulmonary tuberculosis has also been radically modified. In the 1943 edition of Cecil's *Textbook of Medicine*, it is noted that: "The chief principle (of treatment) is rest, which may vary from strict rest in bed to a combination of rest periods and regulated exercise. The effect of rest is both local and general. Diminution of the respiratory rate and amplitude implies lessened motion of the lung which is known to favor healing of tuberculous lesions."[7] Strümpell, in his *Textbook of Internal Medicine* (1929 edition), recommends that tuberculous patients should spend the greater part of the day in the open air on comfortable lounge chairs. "Thereby any unnecessary exertion, any stress on the respiratory system and any irritation on the respiratory passages is avoided. The dissipation of body heat, facilitated by the open air, stimulates the metabolism. Moderate activity in the open air will not be harmful to many patients and is perhaps beneficial. However, even with a minimal temperature elevation absolute bed rest is mandatory."[8] It is interesting that these authors were not only content to prescribe what was the accepted form of therapy of the time, but also searched for physiologic underpinnings to support the rest treatment of tuberculosis.

The rest cure of tuberculosis created a virtual industry. Especially in the mountainous regions of central Europe, numerous sanatoria for patients with tuberculosis were established, and often the patients stayed there for months or years, subjected to a rigid routine of open-air cures and regulated activity. Thomas Mann, in his novel *The Magic Mountain*, has described how life in such an isolated and somewhat artificial community leads to demoralization and personality disintegration. With the advent of chemotherapy, the rest-cure treatment of pulmonary tuberculosis has all but disappeared. Patients can now be treated while ambulatory with relatively little disruption of their personal lives.

Another revolution has occurred in the management of postoperative patients. After almost any type of operation patients remained in bed for many days or weeks. The postoperative morbidity, constipation, urinary retention, and weakness were often due to the prolonged immobilization, rather than to the operation. In 1944, Powers published the results of a controlled study in which he demonstrated that early ambulation greatly reduced the postoperative morbidity.[9] This concept was quickly accepted. Early ambulation not only has made for a more rapid recovery, but by reducing the number of hospital days it has cut the cost of care. After an uncomplicated herniorrhaphy a patient will now be discharged in 3 to 5 days. Before Powers' report patients remained in the hospital for 2 weeks.

In the following chapters, the effects of immobilization on circulation and respiration, bone, muscle, joints, and skin and on the emotional and intellectual capabilities will be explored in detail. These effects, as will be demonstrated, can be profound. When immobilization is forced upon an individual by nature of disease or injury, its potential deleterious effects must be recognized and corrective measures taken whenever possible. As a form of therapy bed rest may be beneficial or harmful. It can be used to the patient's advantage or it can be abused. As for all potent remedies, the degree and duration of bed confinement must be carefully prescribed, keeping in mind its harmful aspects. R. A. J. Asher, in a discussion on "Dangers of Going to Bed," aptly paraphrased a verse by Bishop Thomas Ken[10]:

> Teach us to live that we may dread
> Unnecessary time in bed.
> Get people up and we may save
> Our patients from an early grave.

REFERENCES

1. Andersen, K. L., Shephard, R. J., Denolin, H., Varnauskas, E.; and Masironi, R. *Fundamentals of Exercise Testing.* Geneva, 1971. World Health Organization.
2. Browse, N. L. *The Physiology and Pathology of Bed Rest.* Springfield, 1965. Charles C. Thomas.
3. Deitrick, J. E., Whedon, G. D., and Shorr, E. Effects of immobilization upon various metabolic and physiologic functions of normal men. *Am. J. Med.* 4:3, 1948.
4. Spencer, W. A., Vallbona, C., and Carter, R. E. Physiologic concepts of immobilization. *Arch. Phys. Med. Rehab.* 46:89, 1965.
5. Levine, S. A. *Clinical Heart Disease.* 5th Ed. Philadelphia, 1958. W. B. Saunders.
6. Zeller, J. W., Waine, H., and Jellinek, K. Sanatorium management of rheumatoid arthritis. *J. Am. Med. Assoc.* 186:1143, 1963.
7. Cecil, R. L. *A Textbook of Medicine.* 6th Ed. Philadelphia, 1943. W. B. Saunders.
8. Strümpell, A., and Seyfarth, C. *Lehrbuch der Speziellen Pathologie und Therapie der Inneren Krankheiten.* 28th Ed. Leipzig, 1929. F. C. W. Vogel.
9. Powers, J. H. The abuse of rest as a therapeutic measure in surgery. *J. Am. Med. Assoc.* 125:1079, 1944.
10. Asher, R. A. J. Dangers of going to bed. *Br. Med. J.* 2:967, 1947.

CHAPTER 2

The Effects of Immobilization on Circulation and Respiration

Any individual who has spent several days in bed has experienced the deconditioning effect caused by prolonged bed rest. When first resuming an upright position, the heart pounds, the head feels drained of blood, the skin becomes moist with sweat, and fainting is not uncommon. The patient feels weak with a diminished tolerance to exertion. One of the major advances in medical care during World War II was the institution of early ambulation after illness and surgical operations. The period of bed rest after repairs of hernias, for instance, was reduced from 2 weeks to a few days. Early ambulation drastically reduced the morbidity of surgical procedures which, as it turned out, had been due to immobilization as much as to the procedures themselves.

Deitrick, Whedon, and Shorr were among the first to study the effect of immobilization on various physiologic functions of normal men.[1] Four healthy men were immobilized for 6 to 7 weeks by bed rest, enforced by the application of a body plaster cast. Within a week of the institution of immobilization, the subjects developed an increasing tendency to fainting when tilted to an erect position. This tendency became more pronounced as the period of immobilization

11

advanced. Fainting was closely correlated with the decrease of the pulse pressure. It occurred when the pulse pressure reached the critically low level of 10 to 12 mm Hg. An extensive study of the effects of prolonged bed rest on cardiovascular and pulmonary functions was conducted by Saltin and co-workers[2] in 1968. Their observations were made on five healthy young men who were subjected to 20 days of complete bed rest followed by a period of intensive physical training. We owe much of our knowledge on the debilitating effect of immobilization to Saltin's thorough investigation.

CARDIOVASCULAR FUNCTION AT REST

Resting Heart Rate.   Deitrick *et al.*[1] reported an increase of the resting heart rate during immobilization averaging 3.8 beats/min. During the first 3 weeks of recovery, there was a further increase which averaged 4.7 beats/min. Thereafter, the heart rate decreased to the control level. Saltin and co-workers[2] computed the basal heart rate during 20 days of bed rest from 7 to 8 hr of continuous tape recordings. The resting heart rate increased during the period of immobilization by 0.4 beats/min/day.

Resting Blood Pressure.   Both Deitrick[1] and Saltin[2] reported that prolonged bed rest did not alter the arterial blood pressure. Sokoll *et al.,*[3] however, found a significant fall in the resting systolic pressure after 3 weeks of bed rest. There was no change in the diastolic pressure.

Heart Volume.   Twenty days of bed rest reduced the heart volume by 11 percent as measured by radiographic techniques. Physical training for 13 to 15 days after the period of bed rest restored the heart volume to its original value.[2]

Stroke Volume. Bed rest lowered the stroke volume by 16 percent when measured in the supine position. The decrease was substantially greater when the stroke volume was determined in the sitting position.[2]

Cardiac Output. In general the cardiac output is lower when determined in the sitting rather than in the supine position. This differential was not significantly affected by prolonged bed rest.

Blood Volume. Saltin observed an average decrease of the total blood volume by 7 percent during 20 days of bed rest. The plasma volume was proportionally more reduced than the red cell mass.

These findings are by and large in agreement with data obtained by Miller,[4] Johnson,[5] and Vogt.[6] Greenleaf *et al.*[7] reported that 4 days of bed rest decreased the plasma volume by 12.6 percent. During the same period of time, the total extracellular fluid volume had decreased by 4.4 percent. It is of interest that by the 13th day of bed rest, the extracellular fluid volume had been restored, while the plasma volume had continued to fall. Apparently the preservation of the extracellular fluid compartment as a whole takes precedence over the maintenance of the plasma volume. Isometric and isotonic exercises performed during bed rest reduce the loss of the extracellular fluid and plasma volumes.

THE EFFECT OF BED REST ON EXERCISE TOLERANCE

The most sensitive index of physical fitness is the oxygen uptake during maximal exercise. Saltin[2] reported that after 20 days of bed rest the maximal oxygen uptake had declined by 27 percent, from an average of 3.3 liters/min to 2.4 liters/min. These findings are in agreement with data obtained by other investigators.[8-10] The weight of evidence, therefore, supports the view that prolonged immobilization has an adverse effect on physical fitness as measured by the response to maximal exercise. It is of interest that the decline of maximal oxygen uptake was almost as great when exercise testing was performed in the supine as in the upright position. The decrease of the maximal oxygen uptake after immobilization was due to a reduction of the stroke volume, and the maximal heart rate remained unchanged.

During submaximal exercise the heart rate corresponding to a given oxygen uptake was markedly increased. For instance, work requiring an oxygen cost of 2 liters/min was performed with a heart rate of 145 beats/min before bed rest. After 20 days of bed rest, the heart rate at the same level of oxygen uptake had risen to 180 beats/min. At an exercise load of 600 kpm/min, the heart rate was 129 beats/min before and 154 beats/min after bed rest.

A number of methods have been devised which allow the estimation of maximal oxygen uptake from data obtained during submaximal exercise.[11] Chase *et al.*, however, have pointed out that bed rest alters the relationship of submaximal exercise heart rate to maximal oxygen uptake and maximal work capacity to an extent that makes such extrapolations invalid.[12]

Bed rest lowers the stroke volume during submaximal exercise. In Saltin's study the stroke volume fell from 113 ml before to 92 ml after bed rest at an exercise intensity of 300 kpm/min performed in the supine position. For an exercise intensity of 600 kpm/min the respective data were 116 ml and 89 ml. The cardiac output, which is the product of stroke volume and heart rate, at 300 kpm/min exercise was only slightly lowered by bed rest. The decrease was somewhat greater at 600 kpm/min exercise. The effect of immobilization on cardiovascular function is summarized in Figure 1.

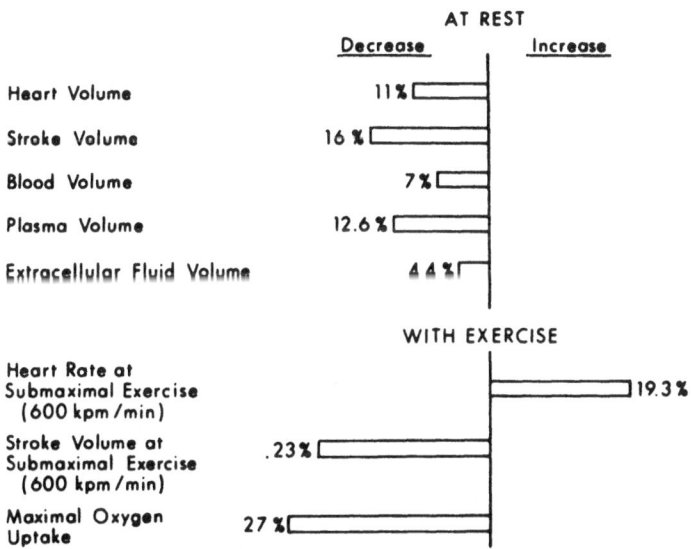

FIGURE 1. Effect of immobilization on cardiovascular function.

Saltin emphasizes that the tolerance to both supine and upright exercise deteriorates equally after extended bed rest. From this he concludes that a diminution of myocardial performance, rather than orthostatic intolerance, may be the most important factor in reducing effort tolerance during immobilization. This assumption is supported by the findings of Sokoll et al., who reported that 3 weeks of bed rest reduced the ventricular ejection time and duration of the diastole.[3] The electrocardiogram showed changes compatible with left ventricular preponderance. In addition, a reduction of the venomotor tone and a so far poorly understood alteration of oxygen utilization by the peripheral tissues may also play important roles in the deconditioning brought about by prolonged immobilization.

The immobilization of patients after injuries or orthopedic and other surgical procedures may be unavoidable.

For better medical care it is important to know if exercise
performed during immobilization will decrease or prevent
deconditioning. This problem has not been extensively investigated. Bassey *et al.* studied 26 males who had undergone knee surgery.[13] Some of the patients were kept at strict
rest for 2 weeks while others were immobilized for only 4
days and then allowed to ambulate. Another subgroup received daily physical therapy while on 2 weeks of bed rest.
The patients on strict bed rest had a distinctly higher heart
rate on submaximal exercise testing for a given oxygen consumption than before surgery. This aspect of deconditioning
was prevented by ambulation or physical therapy. The patients on complete bed rest had a lower systolic blood pressure for a given heart rate during exercise testing when compared to the preoperative response. Stremel and co-workers
placed seven healthy young men on three 2-week periods of
strict bed rest separated by 3-week ambulatory recovery
periods.[10] During one bed rest period no exercise was given.
During one period the individuals performed static exercise
at 21 percent of maximal leg extension. During another bedrest period dynamic exercises were done at 68 percent of
V_{O_2max}. All exercises were performed in the supine position
for 30 min twice a day. The static exercise was intermittent;
each minute of effort was followed by one minute of rest.
During the no-exercise period, V_{O_2max} declined by 12.3 percent and during the dynamic exercise phase by 9.2 percent,
but during the static exercise period by only 4.8 percent. The
maximal heart rate increased during all three excercise regimes. At submaximal workloads the oxygen uptake per
given workload declined during all three exercise regimes.
The reduction was less marked during the static exercise
phase. The apparent advantage of static over dynamic exercise is offset by the observation that the reduction of the

plasma volume during bed rest is the least in the dynamic exercise period. This finding was confirmed by later observations from the same laboratory.[7] From these studies one may conclude that a judicious combination of static and dynamic exercises performed during a period of prolonged bed rest may be the most effective means of preventing deconditioning. Chase *et al.*, who tested various excercise regimes during bed rest, found that trampoline activities were the most effective.[12] For obvious reasons this is impractical in a clinical setting.

ORTHOSTATIC TOLERANCE

Even a few days in bed may cause dizziness and faintness when the patient first assumes the upright position. The ability of the circulation to adapt to a sudden shift from the supine to an upright position varies from individual to individual. Immobile standing for any length of time requires an even greater adaptation, which is impaired by a preceding period of immobilization. Orthostatic tolerance is best studied by tilt-table tests. In a normally active individual, the heart rate rises and the blood pressure falls during immobile standing on the tilt table. After immobilization this response is exaggerated. In Deitrick's study fainting occurred when the pulse pressure had fallen to 10–12 mm Hg.[1] Miller *et al.* investigated the orthostatic tolerance of 12 healthy young men who had been subjected to 4 weeks of strict bed rest.[4] They found that the response to tilt-table testing varied from day to day. Therefore, a large number of tilt-table tests were done on each individual in order to minimize the effect of daily variations. Forty-two percent of the individuals did not faint at any time during repeated testing. However, in almost all subjects the highest obtained heart rates during tilting were distinctly greater after than before bed rest. This differential was eliminated when an antigravity suit was worn during tilting.

The mechanism by which bed rest induces orthostatic intolerance is not fully understood. The correlation with the decrease of blood volume is poor.[4,8] Saltin has emphasized that the circulatory response of the immobilized normal individual is different from that of a patient with idiopathic postural hypotension.[2] The patient with orthostatic hypotension caused by central nervous system disease shows an impaired control of resistance and capacitance vessels in the upright position. Saltin was unable to demonstrate the same lack of control in the normal immobilized individual. On the other hand, the patient with idiopathic postural hypotension exhibits a normal circulatory adaptation to muscular exercise as long as he or she is in the supine position. As described earlier in this chapter, this is not the case for the individual who has been immobilized for a period of time. Hyatt et al. studied the orthostatic response of 12 healthy young individuals before and after 2 weeks of strict bed rest.[14] Postrecumbency tilting resulted in a more marked increase of the heart rate and in a more distinct decrease of stroke volume and cardiac output. Bed rest caused an extensive diuresis of water and sodium, leading to a net water loss of 3 liters in 2 weeks. Both plasma and extracellular fluid volume fell during the first few days. At the end of the 2-week period, however, the plasma volume had been restored while the interstitial volume had remained low. On the basis of these findings the authors suggest an interesting hypothesis for the pathogenesis of postrecumbency orthostatic intolerance. Recumbency stimulates the low pressure baroceptors in the chest. These centers, in turn, inhibit antidiuretic hormone and aldosterone secretion, resulting in a water and salt diuresis. The dehydration of the extracellular fluid compartment lowers the tissue pressure and decreases the resistance to capillary filtration. Therefore, when an individual is tilted after a period of recumbency, more fluid than normal is filtered from the capillaries into the dehydrated extracellular space. This effect reduces the venous return to the heart and lowers central blood volume and stroke volume. In response, baroceptors increase the heart rate and vasoconstriction. However, the vasoconstriction further compromises the peripheral blood flow and the return of blood to the heart. Eventually vasodilation must supersede in order to maintain a minimal peripheral blood flow. The individual faints when these compensatory mechanisms fail and when the blood pressure has fallen below a critical level. In a subsequent double-blind study the same authors found that the administration of 9-alpha-fluorohydrocortisone minimized the water and sodium diuresis and the reduction of the plasma volume.[15] The heart-rate response to tilt remained unaffected by bed rest in those individuals who received the mineral corticoid. Heart-rate response to excercise and the recovery after excercise were almost indentical before and after bed rest in those who received 9-alpha-fluorohydrocortisone. These results support the assumption that water loss may be at least partly responsible for the orthostatic intolerance that develops after bed rest. Pertinent in this connection are Abelmann's observations that patients in congestive heart failure with increased ventricular filling pressure and central blood volume have a better than normal tolerance to immobile standing.[16] It should be pointed out that Hyatt's hypothesis has been jeopardized by Greenleaf's recent and well-documented observation that after 2 weeks of bed rest, the extracellular interstitial fluid volume had been restored to the original value.[7] Greenleaf's results are at variance with earlier studies[17,18] that detailed a continuing diminution of the extracellular compartment during several weeks of recumbency. Further studies may elucidate these contradictory results.

The weightless state of space travel has sparked a renewed interest in orthostatic intolerance. It presents less of a problem in clinical medicine. Early ambulation has reduced the periods of strict bed rest to a minimum. When a patient has been in bed for a prolonged period of time, syncopal attacks can be minimized by a gradual return to an upright position. The patient should sit on the edge of the bed for a while before being permitted to stand or move to a chair. Elastic stockings or abdominal binders help to prevent the effects of prolonged recumbency.

Orthostatic hypotension is more bothersome in paraplegic and, especially, quadriplegic patients who for various reasons, such as decubitus ulcer care or tong traction, had to remain recumbent for some time. The hypotensive episodes continue for some time and simple measures, such as elastic stockings or abdominal binders, may not be effective. There is some evidence that adrenocortical functions are altered in patients with spinal cord lesions. Kaplan *et al.* reported that approximately 60 percent of their patients with spinal-cord injury did not increase the 17-ketosteroid and 17-hydroxy-steroid excretion in response to the administration of ACTH.[19] Vallbona and co-workers showed that quadriplegic patients who became hypotensive on passive tilt showed no increase of the plasma cortisol concentration in contrast to normal individuals who also had a hypotensive response to tilting.[20] Quadriplegic patients excreted more than three times the normal amount of corticoids in the urine. The authors conclude from this observation that the quadriplegic patient is in a state of chronic stress which may have led to relative adrenocortical exhaustion and an inability to respond to the newly superimposed stress of tilting with more cortisol production. The authors recommend the administration of an adrenocorticoid to quadriplegic patients who present with severe persistent hypotensive responses on assuming an upright position.

Venous Thrombosis

The formation of blood clots in the veins of the lower extremities and pelvis is a well-known risk of prolonged immobilization. In 1862, Virchow postulated that three factors had to interact to cause a thrombosis in a vein: a change in the rate of blood flow, changes in the vessel wall, and a change in the coagulability of the blood. More than 100 years later, the precise role of each of these three factors is still not fully understood. There is no clear-cut evidence at this point in time that prolonged bed rest by itself, without other contributing factors, predisposes to the development of venous thrombosis. Early studies have shown that the velocity of blood flow in the lower extremity veins is actually greater in the recumbent position than in standing or sitting. Eighteen days of bed rest did not slow the ankle-to-groin venous flow time.[21] There is no proof, therefore, that bed rest by itself causes a stasis in the veins of the lower extremities. Even the relationship of stasis to intravascular clotting is not clear. In Wessler's experiments it took 8 hr before blood trapped between two ligatures of a dog's vein was fully coagulated.[22] Clearly, factors other than the immobilization alone must play a part in enhancing the risk of thrombosis during prolonged bed rest.

Sevitt and Gallagher[23] found deep vein thromboses in

65 percent of autopsies of 125 patients who had died following injuries and burns. Patients with pulmonary emboli were
excluded from this series. The incidence of thrombosis increased with the lengthening of the survival time. This might
suggest a direct relationship of the length of bed rest to the
development of thrombi. However, no general conclusions
can be drawn from this select group of patients who had
come to autopsy. Furthermore, in the presence of severe
injury, factors other than bed rest may have contributed
more significantly to the incidence of thrombosis and its increase with the length of survival. In a more recent study, 53
percent of 76 patients with stroke developed a deep venous
thrombosis in the paralyzed leg, as detected by the [^{125}I]fi-
brinogen technique. Only 5 patients had a thrombosis of the
nonparalyzed leg.[24] The authors searched for predisposing
factors. A statistically significant relationship was established only with the presence of varicose veins and only in
the normal limb. A history of previous thromboembolism,
the presence or abscence of voluntary motion in the hemiplegic limb, an increase or decrease of muscle tone, and
coexisting heart failure or atrial fibrillation bore no relationship to the incidence of venous thrombosis. The number of
days for which patients were confined to bed also did not
affect the incidence of deep vein thrombosis. Those who
were allowed up after 4 days had the same incidence as those
patients who remained in bed for 10 days or longer. Also, the
fact that the incidence was much lower in the nonparalyzed
than in the paralyzed leg suggests that bed rest as such is not
an important factor. In a study of chronic rather than acute
hemiplegia 33 percent of 150 patients had developed a
thrombosis in the paralyzed limb as demonstrated by venography.[25] The incidence increased with the degree of paralysis
of the hemiplegic leg. Warlow *et al.* conclude that "probably

the early onset of deep vein thrombosis, detected with [^{125}I]fibrinogen, in patients who have been acutely ill is independent of the period of confinement to bed, whereas the subsequent propagation and embolization of thrombi, as detected by necropsy, may not be."[24]

If immobilization were an important cause of phlebothrombosis, a high incidence should be expected throughout the lifetime of paraplegic patients. Bors found deep vein thrombosis by venography in 58 of 99 paraplegic patients.[26] Watson reported an incidence of venous thrombosis of 12.5 percent in 431 paraplegic and quadriplegic patients.[27] The rate was highest for patients with lesions of the thoracic spine. Watson and other British workers reported that the incidence was the highest within 2 months after injury and declined thereafter. This again suggests that factors other than immobilization must play a role. This contention is supported by Naso's report that the blood in three out of six patients with acute spinal cord injury showed evidence of hypercoagulability, either by an increase of factor VIII or by a shortened platelet survival.[28]

Virchow's second factor, changes in the intima of the vein, may contribute to phlebothromboses in immobilized patients. Veins may be kinked by awkward positioning, causing endothelial damage. The Fowler's position, now rarely used, in which the knees are flexed over a rigid support, may cause damage to the popliteal vein as pointed out by Browse.[29] The compression of one calf by the tibial crest of the other leg may have the same effect. Even a small area of intimal injury may serve as a nidus to which platelets may adhere and where thrombus formation might begin.

A change in the coagulability of the blood may be the most salient factor in the genesis of venous thrombosis. A detailed discussion of this aspect is beyond the scope of this chapter. However, elevations in the plasma procoagulants and fibrinogen and an increase in the number and reactivity of platelets and changes in fibrinolysis are common after surgical operations and injuries.[30] Within a span of 4 months, Micheli encountered thromboembolic complications in six active and fairly young patients who had one extremity immobilized in a plaster cast for the treatment of a fracture.[31] Medical illness, especially when associated with prolonged bed rest and advanced age and obesity, predisposes to thromboembolic complications. The association of venous thrombosis with certain tumors, such as carcinoma of the tail of the pancreas or of the lung, is well known. The underlying disease or trauma which may change blood coagulability is probably more important than the immobilization that accompanies the treatment of the disease. Lorentsen *et al.* found no evidence of hypercoagulability in 12 elderly patients who were bedridden because of advanced senility but who had no demonstrably significant medical illness.[32] In this connection the observations of Murray *et al.* are also significant.[33] Of 35 patients treated for myocardial infarction, 12 developed deep vein thromboses, 10 of them within the first few days of illness. On the other hand, of 15 patients with the suspected diagnosis of myocardial infarction, which eventually proved to be erroneous, only one developed a deep vein thrombosis even though these patients underwent the same treatment as the myocardial infarction group including strict bed rest. Immobilization is just one and apparently not the most important factor in the pathogenesis of thromboembolic complications in patients who are put to bed following injury, surgical operations, and medical illness.

The prevention of postoperative and posttraumatic lower extremity thrombosis is important since pulmonary emboli constitute a major cause of postoperative mortality. Since 50–80 percent of pulmonary emboli occur in patients in whom the presence of leg vein thrombosis had remained undetected, the emphasis should be on prevention rather than on treatment of established phlebothrombosis. The prophylactic use of anticoagulants in certain high-risk patients is now well accepted. The use of low-dose heparin and of drugs which reduce platelet aggregation, such as aspirin and dipyridamole, carries fewer risks than anticoagulation, but their value in the prevention of venous thrombosis has not been well established.[30]

Physical measures that accelerate the blood flow in the veins reduce the incidence of clot formation. As pointed out before, prolonged bed rest does not lower the velocity of blood flow through lower extremity veins. On the other hand it stands to reason that blood that flows more rapidly is less likely to clot, regardless of other circumstances. Therefore, patients should be taught how to exercise their lower extremity muscles. The use of elastic stockings or bandages has become routine in many institutions. Proper application is important. Husni et al. have shown that elastic bandages across the knee raise the venous pressure in the distal circulation and act as tourniquets.[34] They recommend that elastic bandages should terminate below the knee. Sigel et al. have measured the velocity of flow in lower extremity veins using a Doppler ultrasound technique.[35] Full length elastic stockings increased the velocity of blood flow through the lower extremity veins by 100 percent. After 3 hr of wear the flow velocity was still 80 percent above base line. After removal of the stocking the velocity remained elevated for another 30 min. The elastic compression also diminished the waxing and waning effect of respiration on the venous blood flow and made it more even. This study indicates that properly applied full-length elastic stockings accelerate the flow-through veins and may indeed contribute significantly to the prevention of thromboses. Elevation of the legs also increases venous blood-flow velocity. In Sigel's study, body tilt to a foot-up position increased the venous blood flow velocity by 30 percent. If for any reason elastic stockings cannot be worn, the patient should be positioned with the feet slightly elevated.

RESPIRATION

In years past a terminal pneumonia has frequently been the dreaded outcome of a long illness that had confined a patient to bed for extended periods of time. Today, early mobilization, respiratory care, and antibiotic therapy have reduced the incidence and import of ventilatory insufficiency and respiratory infection that may follow serious illness or trauma. Nevertheless, the combination of illness, debility, and immobility continues to be a significant risk for the development of potentially fatal respiratory infections. Which of these factors is the most important it is impossible to say. It is certainly true that the immobilized healthy individual will not develop pneumonia. On the other hand, in the infirm ill patient the incidence of pneumonia can be greatly reduced by prophylactic measures which assure efficient ventilation of all segments of the lungs.

Even through generations of physicians have dreaded pneumonia as a complication of prolonged bed rest, the subject has received little attention by investigators. Saltin reported that prolonged strict immobilization of healthy men produced no changes in pulmonary function.[2] Specifically, total lung capacity, forced vital capacity, forced expiratory volume, alveolar–arterial oxygen tension difference, and membrane diffusing capacity remained unchanged. When exercise was performed during the period of bed rest, the tidal volume was lower and the respiratory rate higher than during the control phase. The ventilatory equivalent (the ratio of minute volume of respiration to oxygen uptake) was not affected by bed rest. Earlier, Deitrick et al. had arrived at similar results.[1]

The mechanics of air exchange, therefore, appear to be little affected by immobility, but there are other factors which predispose to respiratory infections. Browse has pointed out that the supine position interferes with the efficiency of the cilia, which under normal conditions sweep mucus from the small through the larger bronchi to the trachea and larynx.[29] In the upright position the bronchioles run vertically in a cephalad direction and their epithelium is covered by a thin, even layer of mucus. In a supine body position the same bronchioles are horizontal. Gravity now makes the mucus form a puddle on the lower side of the bronchiole, while the upper wall loses its covering of mucus, with the result that the epithelium becomes dry and cracks. Both the excessive pooling of mucus on the bottom and the desiccation of the mucous membrane on the top interfere with the cleansing action of the cilia and prepare the soil for bacterial invasion. Because of the anatomic structure of the bronchial tree, the lower lobe bronchi are most vulnerable to the changes just described, and indeed hypostatic pneumonia occurs most frequently in the lower lobes.

In 1942, Berggren demonstrated that the P_{O_2} of the arterial blood declined and arteriovenous shunting increased in immobilized healthy men.[36] This aspect has been again investigated more recently. Ray et al. immobilized dogs in a side-lying position.[37] The pulmonary venous oxygen pressure of the lung underneath dropped rapidly to anoxic levels while it remained high in the upper lung. Arteriovenous shunting appeared within 4 hr and increased rapidly. If, on the other hand, the dogs were turned every half hour, the pulmonary venous oxygen tension shifted back to normal with changes of position, and no shunting occurred. Similar observations were made on two patients who, in addition, had been overhydrated inadvertently. Frequent turning greatly reduced arteriovenous shunting. The importance of this observation is obvious. The dependent pulmonary segments of immobilized patients are poorly ventilated, while blood perfusion continues at a normal rate. The distortion of the ventilation/blood flow ratio leads to increasing degrees of arteriovenous shunting, resulting eventually in arterial hypoxemia. Turning the patient from supine to lateral to prone to supine, at least once per hour, will largely prevent the risks of the ventilation/perfusion imbalance and of arteriovenous shunting.

In addition, the elimination of excessive secretions and the maintenance of patent airways are of utmost importance. The patient should be instructed how to cough effectively. Positional drainage and chest physical therapy should be employed, if needed, around the clock. The room air should be suitably humidified. Suctioning needs to be instituted if the patient is too weak to expectorate excessive secretions. A tracheostomy may be life saving if it becomes important to bypass the upper airways.

The immobilized, obtunded, and weak patient is always at risk of aspirating food or liquids. A circumspect nurse will quickly discover the best position for eating in which the patient is least apt to choke. Many patients can swallow soft food better than liquids. When this presents a problem, fluids may have to be given parenterally while the feeding of high caloric soft foods may continue. Except in neurologic lesions in which the deglutition reflex is affected, this problem is usually resolved once the patient is able to get up and eat and drink in the sitting position.

SUMMARY

The preceding paragraphs reiterate the dangers of immobilization and its deleterious effects on the vital functions of circulation and respiration. The efficiency of the human body as a whole is enhanced by motion and frequent shifts of position. During immobilization the stroke volume of the heart is reduced while the heart rate accelerates. The ability to adapt to physical effort diminishes rapidly, and, depending upon the length of immobility, days or weeks of conditioning exercises are needed before the efficiency and adaptability have been restored. The ability to accommodate to the upright position is diminished by just a few days of bed rest. An investigation of the orthostatic intolerance of immobilization has shown that it is accompanied by profound changes in water and salt metabolism and by a significant loss of plasma and extracellular compartment volumes. As far as respirations are concerned, the ability of the bronchial tree to rid itself of foreign material and of excess mucus is very much affected. Furthermore, immobilization in the same position interferes precariously with the balance of ventilation and pulmonary circulation, causing a physiologic arteriovenous shunt and arterial anoxia. A simple maneuver such as turning the patient every hour will eliminate this risk.
The dangers of immobility have been known to physicians for a long time. Over the last 30 years physiologic measurements have helped to explain the mechanisms underly-

ing the risks of immobility and have provided a scientific
base for well-known and long-established clinical facts.

REFERENCES

1. Deitrick, J. E., Whedon, G. D., and Shorr, E. Effects of immobilization
   upon various metabolic and physiologic functions of normal men. *Am.
   J. Med.* **4**:3, 1948.
2. Saltin, B. Blomqvist, G., Mitchell, J. H., Johnson, R. L., Wilden-
   thal, K., and Chapman, C. B. Response to exercise after bed rest and
   after training. *Circulation* **38**(Suppl. VII):1, 1968.
3. Sokol, U., Kessel, R., and Lang, E. Auswirkungen einer laengeren
   Immobilisation auf die Herz—and Kreislaufdynamik. *Muench. Med.
   Wochenschr.* **115**:69, 1973.
4. Miller, P. B., Johnson, R. L., and Lamb, L. E. Effects of four weeks of
   absolute bed rest on circulatory functions in man. *Aerosp. Med.*
   35:1194, 1964.
5. Johnson, P. C., Driscoli, T. B., and Carpentier, W. R. Vascular and
   extravascular fluid changes during six days of bed rest. *Aerosp. Med.*
   42:875, 1971.
6. Vogt, F. B., Mack, P. B., and Johnson, P. C. Tilt table response and
   blood volume changes associated with thirty days of recumbency.
   Aerosp. Med. **37**:771, 1966.
7. Greenleaf, J. E., Bernauer, E. M., Young, H. L., Morse, J. T., Staley,
   R. W., Juhos, L. T., and Van Beaumont, W. Fluid and electrolyte shifts
   during bed rest with isometric and isotonic exercise. *J. Appl. Physiol.*
   42:59, 1977.
8. Taylor, H. L., Henschel, A., Brozek, J., and Keys, A. Effects of bed
   rest on cardiovascular function and work performance. *J. Appl.
   Physiol.* **2**:223, 1949.
9. Miller, P. B., Johnson, R. L., and Lamb, L. E. Effects of moderate
   physical exercise during four weeks of bed rest on circulatory
   functions in man *Aerosp. Med.* **36**:1077, 1965.
10. Stremel, R. W., Convertino, V. A., Bernauer, E. M., and Greenleaf, J.
    E. Cardiorespiratory deconditioning with static and dynamic leg exer-
    cise during bed rest. *J. Appl. Physiol.* **41**:905, 1976.
11. Astrand, P. O. and Ryhming, I. A nomogram for calculation of
    aerobic capacity (physical fitness) from pulse rate during submaximal
    work. *J. Appl. Physiol.* **7**:218, 1954.

12. Chase, G. A., Grave, C., and Rowell, L. B. Independence of changes in functional and performance capacities attending prolonged bed rest. *Aerosp. Med.* **37**:1232, 1966.
13. Bassey, E. J., Bennett, T., Birmingham, A. T., Fentem, P. H., Fitton, D., and Goldsmith, R. Effects of surgical operation and bed rest on cardiovascular responses to exercise in hospital patients. *Cardiovasc. Res.* **7**:588, 1973.
14. Hyatt, K. H., Kamenetsky, L. G., and Smith, W. M. Extravascular dehydration as an etiologic factor in post-recumbency orthostatism. *Aerosp. Med.* **40**:644, 1969.
15. Bohnn, B. J., Hyatt, K. H., Kamenetsky, L. G., Calder, B. E., and Smith, W. M. Prevention of bed rest induced orthostatism by 9-alpha-fluorohydrocortisone. *Aerosp. Med.* **41**:495, 1970.
16. Abelmann, W. H. and Fareeduddin, K. Increased tolerance or orthostatic stress in patients with heart disease. *Am. J. Cardiol.* **23**:354, 1969.
17. White, P. D., Nyberg, J. W., Finney, L. M., and White, W. J. A comparative study of the physiological effects of immersion and bed rest. Douglas Aircraft Corp. Report DAC-59226, 1966.
18. Vogt, F. B. and Johnson, P. C. Plasma volume and extracellular fluid volume change associated with 10 days of bed recumbency. *Aerosp. Med.* **38**:21, 1967.
19. Kaplan, L., Powell, B. R., Grynbaum, B. B., and Rusk, H. A. Comprehensive follow-up study of spinal cord dysfunction and its resultant disabilities. *Institute of Rehabilitation Medicine*, p. 63. New York, 1966. New York University Medical Center.
20. Vallbona, C., Lipscomb, H. S., and Carter, R. E. Endocrine responses to orthostatic hypotension in quadriplegia. *Arch. Phys. Med. Rehab.* **47**:412, 1966.
21. Wright, H. P., Osborn, S. B., and Hayden, M. Venous velocity in bedridden medical patients. *Lancet* **2**:699, 1952.
22. Wessler, S. Studies in intravascular coagulation. I. Coagulation in isolated venous segments. *J. Clin. Invest.* **31**:1011, 1952.
23. Sevitt, S. and Gallagher, N. Venous thrombosis and pulmonary embolism *Br. J. Surg.* **48**:475, 1961.
24. Warlow, C., Ogston, D., and Douglas, A. S. Deep venous thrombosis of legs after strokes. Part I—Incidence and predisposing factors. *Br. Med. J.* **1**:1178, 1976.
25. Cope, C., Reyes, T. M., and Skversky, N. J. Phlebographic analysis of the incidence of thrombosis in hemiplegia. *Radiology* **109**:581, 1973.
26. Bors, E., Conrad, C. A., and Massell, T. B. Venous occlusion of lower extremities in paraplegic patients. *Surg. Gynecol. Obstet.* **99**:451, 1954.

27. Watson, N. Venous thrombosis and pulmonary embolism in spinal cord injury. *Paraplegia* **6**:113, 1968/1969.
28. Naso, F. Pulmonary embolism in acute spinal cord injury. *Arch. Phys. Med. Rehab.* **55**:275, 1974.
29. Browse, N. L. *Physiology and Pathology of Bed Rest.* Springfield, Illinois, 1965. Charles C Thomas.
30. Clagett, G. P. and Salzman, E. W. Prevention of venous thromboembolism in surgical patients. *N. Engl. J. Med.* **290**:93, 1974.
31. Micheli, L. J. Thromboembolic complications of cast immobilization for injuries of the lower extremities. *Clin. Orthop.* **108**:191, 1975.
32. Lorentsen, E., Eika, C., and Godal, H. C. Coagulation studies in chronically bedridden patients. *Acta Med. Scand.* **195**:79, 1974.
33. Murray, T. S., Lorimer, A. R., Cox, F. C. and Lawrie, T. D. V. Leg vein thrombosis following myocardial infarction. *Lancet* **2**:792, 1970.
34. Husni, E. A., Ximenes, J. O. C., and Hamilton, F. G. Pressure bandaging of the lower extremity. *J. Am. Med. Assoc.* **206**:2715, 1968.
35. Sigel, B., Edelstein, A. L., Felix, W. R., Jr., and Memhardt, C. R. Compression of the deep venous system of the lower leg during inactive recumbency. *Arch. Surg.* **106**:38, 1973.
36. Berggren, S. M. Oxygen deficit of arterial blood caused by nonventilating parts of the lungs. *Acta Physiol. Scand.* **4**(Suppl. 2):1, 1942.
37. Ray, J. F. III, Yost, L., Moallem, S., Sanoudos, G. M., Villemena, P., Paredes, R. M., and Clauss, R. H. Immobility, hypoxemia and pulmonary arteriovenous shunting. *Arch. Surg.* **109**:537, 1974.

CHAPTER 3

The Effects of Immobilization on Bone

Accretion and resorption of the skeletal mass, especially of the lower part of the body, are maintained in equilibrium by the stimulus of weight bearing and activity. Immobilization, whether by prolonged recumbency, paralysis, or space-flight immobilization, leads to bone atrophy. Calcium released by the immobilized skeleton is excreted in the urine with resulting hypercalciuria ultimately reflecting the extent of bone loss. The excessive elimination of calcium salts in the urine also predisposes to nephrocalcinosis and nephrolithiasis, the latter representing a frequent complication of spinal-cord lesions. The deposition of calcium salts in soft tissues is another sequela of loss of calcium from the skeletal mass.

Immobilization affects organic as well as inorganic constituents of bone. The increased excretion of hydroxyproline during immobilization is evidence that the organic bone matter is being depleted as much as the inorganic mineral components. Immobilization, therefore, leads to a true osteoporosis, since total bone mass decreases with time. Terms such as "decalcification" and "demineralization" do not adequately depict the underlying skeletal lesion.

In addition to the output of calcium salts in the urine,

the degree of bone loss can be assessed by photon beam densitometry, which can detect changes of as little as 2 percent. Radiographs are less sensitive. A bone must have lost at least 40–50 percent of its mineral before the osteopenic process can be detected by routine radiographs. Quantitative histologic examination of bone biopsy specimens and isotope calcium turnover studies represent more sensitive means of detecting the degree of osteopenia produced by immobilization.

Pathology and Pathogenesis

In 1882, von Volkmann reported that injured bones may become diffusely atrophic and demineralized.[1] He named this condition "rarifying osteitis." Von Volkmann further observed that the extent of the atrophy was limited to the injured limb and that the process was rapidly reversed once the bony injury had healed. In subsequent years other observers reported additional cases of posttraumatic bone atrophy and attempted to explain the pathogenesis of this phenomenon. Some theories implicated vasomotor mechanisms while others uggested neurotrophic factors as the cause. In 1908, Legg postulated that inactivity secondary to trauma may by itself be the cause of posttraumatic bone loss.[2] Since then, osteoporosis due to immobilization has become a recognized entity.

A general osteoporosis occurs in individuals who are immobilized by paralysis resulting from neurologic or orthopedic disorders or by prolonged bed rest. A localized osteoporosis is found in injured and immobilized extremities. If a bone is fractured, the osteoporosis involves the entire extremity but is most pronounced in the bones distal to the fracture site. The loss of bone substance is most marked in the cancellous bone of the metaphysis and the epiphysis. The first signs of osteoporosis are found in the epiphyseal subchondral area. From there it extends to include the entire epiphysis, the latter ultimately assuming a moth-eaten appearance. In contrast, the thin calcified layer of bone underneath the joint cartilage appears more prominent and looks as if it had been drawn out with pencil[3] (Figure 2). Somewhat later, the compact cortical bone becomes involved. The osteones are widened and become confluent, giving the bony substance a spongy appearance. The bone marrow space also becomes larger. Cortical atrophy makes its first appearance in the subperiosteal region in contrast to senile osteoporosis which develops from the marrow outward.[4] The hardness of bone decreases steadily with the duration of immobilization, and after 12 weeks it is only 55–60 percent of

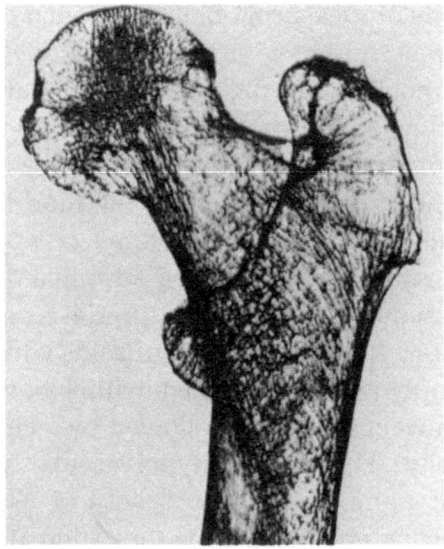

FIGURE 2. Head and neck of femur, osteoporotic due to prolonged immobilization.

normal.[5] At the same time, the elastic resistance of the bone substance increases.

As in all types of osteoporosis, the process must have advanced significantly before it can be demonstrated radiographically. Whedon who studied patients paralyzed by poliomyelitis reported that radiographic evidence of *localized* osteoporosis appeared when 2 percent of the total body calcium had been lost.[6] Osteoporosis first became evident after 3 months of paralysis on the average and first appeared in the proximal and distal ends of the femurs. Osteoporosis of the vertebrae did not become apparent until approximately 10 percent of the total body calcium had been lost.

The development of disuse osteoporosis appears to be linked to the changes in blood flow that occur in immobilized bone. Reports in the literature are contradictory. The picture is confused because different investigators have used different methods of measuring blood flow, have worked with different animals, and have studied the blood flow in various phases of immobilization. Because of the relationship of altered blood flow to the pathogenesis of immobilization osteoporosis, some of the available data will be summarized.

Geiser and Trueta immobilized the hind legs of rabbits by various methods such as tenotomy or application of a plaster cast.[7] Angiographs showed an initial decrease of filling of the osseous blood vessels. After 4–5 days, however, the bone became hypervascular. Sinusoids which previously had been empty were now filled with blood. This phase lasted for 4–6 weeks and was followed by a chronic stage of hypovascularity. During the hypervascular phase an increase in the number of osteoblasts and osteoclasts was noted, suggesting enhanced bone formation and resorption. In the final stage of hypovascularity, both osteoblastic and osteoclastic activity diminished, and the cancellous bone showed no more than a network of thin atrophic trabeculae. Geiser and Trueta's method gave information only on the degree of filling of the vessels. It provided no data on the dynamics of blood flow during immobilization. Hulth and Olerud have reported similar observations.[8] They performed angiographic studies on the legs of rabbits 7 days after they had been immobilized and found dilated and tortuous blood vessels. Sundén studied the blood flow through immobilized bone dynamically by measuring heat clearance from the epiphyseal area.[9] The blood flow increased immediately after motor nerve section and returned to base level after 6 days. He observed an enhanced bone growth during the period of increased blood flow. The point in time in which the heat clearance in Sundén's experiments begins to decrease corresponds to the period when Geiser and Trueta note the onset of hypervascularity. Sundén's findings, therefore, suggest that Geiser and Trueta's period of hypervascularity is associated with a decreased sluggish blood flow. The blood remains stagnant in overfilled vessels.

This concept is further supported by the experiments of Hardt.[10] Ten days after immobilization, he found a decrease of the P_{CO_2} and an increase of the pH and P_{O_2} in the blood of the nutrient vein of bone suggesting an increase of bone blood flow. After 15 days, the condition was reversed. Venous pH and P_{O_2} were now decreased while the P_{CO_2} was increased. At that time the mineral content of the immobilized bone was diminished, compared to the control side. All of these findings taken together suggest that during the early phase of immobilization, the effective blood flow is increased and that bone formation is enhanced. Shortly thereafter the situation is reversed. The effective blood flow is diminished while the blood remains stagnant in overfilled vessels. In this phase bone resorption supervenes.

Little and Valderrama further elaborated on the relationship of immobilization osteoporosis and vascular changes.[11] They described a dilatation of the marrow sinusoids and of the major cortical vascular channels. Osteoclastic activity appeared most pronounced along these widened vessels, suggesting a close correlation between vascular dilatation and osteoclasis. Equilibrium was restored when the process of widening of the vascular channels had reached the outer surface of the bone. At this point the marrow sinusoids returned to their normal state. The cause–effect relationship of hypervascularity to bone resorption remains obscure. Geisei and Trueta[7] have pointed out that it is not logical to regard the hypervascularity as the cause of bone removal because it occurs during both bone formation and destruction.

The factor that is common to all forms of immobilization osteoporosis is lack of muscle activity. Trueta[12] and Valderrama and Trueta[13] examined the effect of muscle contractions on the blood flow in bone by measuring intraosseous pressure. A cannula was threaded into the marrow of dog tibiae and the intramedullary pressure was determined during muscle contractions induced by electrical stimulation and during relaxation. The intramedullary pressure rose during contraction and dropped during the phase of relaxation. The authors concluded that muscle contractions inhibit the venous outflow of blood from bone and force blood to distal unfilled sinusoids. During relaxation the veins empty rapidly, and a suction effect refills the osseous vessels with new arterial blood. Alternating muscle contraction and relaxation therefore promote inflow and outflow of blood to and from bone in a pumplike fashion. When muscle activity ceases, the pumping effect is lost and the venous sinusoids became distended.

Muscle contractions in addition have a direct effect on

bone formation. The pull of contracting muscle produces electric currents in bone with potentials in millivolt magnitudes. The currents, usually designated "piezoelectricity," are proportional to the applied force. Bone regions under mechanical tension act as anodes, compressed regions as cathodes. Bone formation occurs in the cathodal region.[14] The effect of muscle activity on bone mass has been further demonstrated by Doyle et al.[15] They showed in necropsies that the ash weight of the third lumbar vertebra correlated significantly with the weight of the psoas muscle which attaches to it. If it can be assumed that the mass of a muscle corresponds to its force, then it can be concluded that such forces are important factors in bone formation.

Other observations on the effect of experimental immobilization on bone need to be cited. Landry and Fleisch working with rats used the technique of tetracycline staining to measure bone formation.[16] There was an early phase of diminished bone formation which lasted about 12 days. This was followed by a second phase of both increased bone formation and resorption and a third phase of decreased bone formation. Pennock and co-workers found a decrease of ash weight in the femora of rats whose limbs had been immobilized for four weeks.[17] The atrophy was not prevented by calcitonin, a hormone released by the C cells of the thyroid gland, which normally functions to suppress bone resorption. In similar experiments, Mattson described increased anabolic activity and bone formation when the limb was remobilized after 16 weeks of immobilization.[18] However, not all of the lost bone mass was restored. Some of the bone loss remained irreversible.

Uhthoff and Jaworski immobilized one forelimb of young adult beagle dogs by encasing it in plaster.[19] The other forelimb served as a control. Dogs were killed at various points of time, some as early as 2 weeks after immobilization and some as late as 40 weeks. A rapid initial bone loss occurred, reaching its peak at 6 weeks. This was followed by a period of reversal during which the mass of the immobilized bones approached control values. After 12 weeks a second stage of slow but longer-lasting bone loss began which ended 24–32 weeks after immobilization. From then on the bone mass which had been reduced by 30 to 50 percent was maintained at the same level. The distal bones were more affected than the proximal bones. The main loss occurred in the periosteal bone envelope. The periosteal resorption surfaces showed a small increase during the first phase of bone loss and a much higher increase during the second phase.

Burkhart and Jowsey examined the relationship of parathyroid and thyroid hormones to immobilization osteoporosis.[20] They found that, in the dog, osteoporosis developed after 3 weeks of immobilization and reached its peak after 8 weeks. During the period of peak bone resorption the blood of the nutrient osseous vein was acidotic (high P_{CO_2} and low pH) and hypoxic. Removal of the parathyroids before immobilization prevented the development of osteoporosis. Bone formation even in the nonimmobilized limb was further reduced by removal of the thyroid. Apparently the thyroid produces a substance necessary to keep bone tissue responsive to parathyroid hormone. The authors suggest that local factors related to immobilization sensitize bone to circulating parathyroid hormones. Bone under normal mechanical stress appears to be less susceptible to parathyroid hormone and other systemic influences.

Investigations in human immobilized subjects have dealt mostly with calcium balance studies which will be discussed later in this chapter. Heaney, however, explored bone formation and resorption by isotope-kinetic analysis.[21]

He studied patients with immobilization osteoporosis due to poliomyelitis. Six of these patients were in an acute phase of immobilization osteoporosis, that is their calcium balances were still negative. Three additional subjects, in a stable chronic phase, were studied at an average of 7 years after the onset of the paralysis, when their calcium balances were in equilibrium. Control data were obtained on four normal volunteers. In the acute phase, bone formation rates were found to be normal to twice normal while bone resorption rates were two to three times normal. In the stable chronic phase, bone formation and resorption were normal or slightly low. Heaney concluded that the primary mechanism of immobilization osteoporosis was the marked increase of bone resorption, which outweighed bone formation, even though this function was also increased. The observation that bone formation was increased in the acute phase of immobilization osteoporosis conflicted with the time-honored concept that loss of mechanical stress diminishes bone forming activity. Intestinal absorption of calcium was greatly reduced in the acute phase. Treatment with anabolic steroids improved the calcium balance. Kinetic studies showed that this improvement was due to a decrease of bone resorption while bone formation remained unchanged. The equilibrium of bone formation and resorption and of calcium balance in the chronic phase indicates that the process of immobilization osteoporosis is self limiting. An equilibrium is achieved when the total bone mass has been reduced to a certain level. This is in keeping with Willert's observation that immobilization osteoporosis never leads to total bone destruction.[3] He found that in the end stage the number of trabeculae of cancellous bone is diminished but that they may be thickened due to the apposition of new bone, a stage that he called "hypertrophic atrophy."

From a different investigational approach, Minaire and

co-workers arrived at similar results.[22] They performed quantitative histological studies of iliac crest biopsies from 28 immobilized paraplegic patients, combined with metabolic balance measurements. The volume of trabecular bone dropped steadily from its normal value of about 20 percent to a level of 12 percent, which was reached after 25 weeks of immobilization. No further decrease occurred after that time. The periosteocytic lacunae increased in size. The cortices became thinner showing a loss of about 50 percent. The osteoid volume of cancellous bone was decreased by week 10; then it increased again and stabilized at values slightly below normal. Tetracycline staining showed a very significant decrease of the appositional osteoblastic rate. The volume of the adipose tissue and cell population of the marrow showed an early decrease. However, by week 20 it had increased to twice normal values and finally stabilized in a normal range. The authors reported a decrease of the total iliac bone mass at an average of 33 percent. The relative bone loss depends on the bone mass present at the time of immobilization. The greater the preexisting bone mass the greater is the relative loss. In any case, it appears that the trabecular bone volume does not decrease below the level of 12 percent. It stabilizes at this level. The resorption surfaces of cancellous bone were found to increase early, reaching a maximum at 15 weeks, a point in time which coincides with the time of maximum excretion of calcium and hydroxyproline. Since both osteoid volume and calcification appositional rates as determined by tetracycline labeling are low, the authors conclude that the rate of bone apposition is extremely low in immobilization osteoporosis. This is at variance with the conclusions that Heaney reached from his isotope studies.[21]

In summary, the pathogenesis of immobilization osteoporosis is linked to an alteration in the balance of bone formation and resorption. While some observers reported an increase of bone formation in the early phases,[9,10,21] all investigators agree that osteoclastosis and bone resorption are predominant and are primarily responsible for the loss of bone mass. Immobilization osteoporosis is associated with alterations of the blood flow through bone and marrow. Of these, the widening of major vascular channels and marrow sinusoids is most conspicuous. A cause–effect relationship of the changes in blood flow to loss of bone substance has not been established. The process of immobilization osteoporosis is self-limited, and the balance between bone formation and resorption is restored when the bone mass has been reduced to a certain critical level.

LOCALIZED IMMOBILIZATION OSTEOPOROSIS IN MAN

Since von Volkmann's original description,[1] it has become common knowledge that bone of injured or paralyzed extremities becomes demineralized. However, only a few systematic studies are on record. Nilsson[23] studied the mineral mass of the distal femora in 116 patients with fractures of the tibial shaft. Using densitometric methods, he found a mineral loss of 25 percent, compared to the contralateral extremity. The extent of bone loss varied with the severity of the injury and the length of immobilization time. The restoration of bone mass was very slow. In male patients it took several years; in females the pretraumatic state was not restored at all.

A localized osteoporosis in the paralyzed extremities of stroke victims has been reported by a number of observers. Hodkinson and Brain[24] described a significant osteoporosis in the femora of 14 hemiplegic patients. The degree of osteoporosis was determined by measuring the cortical thickness, the sound leg serving as control. Four patients of their series suffered femoral fractures with trivial trauma. The degree of spasticity did not affect the development of osteoporosis. The duration of the paralysis by the time the measurements were made varied from 6 to 105 months.

Panin et al.[25] determined the cortical thickness of humerus, radius, and third metacarpal of 25 hemiplegic upper extremities and compared the results with the sound side. All of the patients had been hemiplegic for at least 6 months. They reported a significant loss of bone mass in all patients. The osteoporosis appeared to be more pronounced in females. It made no difference whether the paralyzed extremity was dominant or nondominant.

The return of motor function decreased the tendency to bone mass loss, but the development of spasticity had no such salutary effect. The authors conclude that "a certain optimal force constellation (degree of force, angle of pull, and torque) may be necessary to prevent or even retard osteoporosis." The authors suggest that this favorable constellation may be provided by voluntary contractions but not by spasticity.

Naftchi and co-workers[26] measured bone demineralization in the forearm of hemiplegic patients. They employed a densitometric method and used the forearm of the sound side as a control. The demineralization was greater in females than in males. The loss of bone density was greater when the hemiplegia had affected the nondominant arm. Since all determinations were expressed as the ratio of the involved to the sound side one can assume that the dominant arm had a greater mineral content than the nondominant side before the patient was struck with paralysis. Approximately 3 months after the stroke the average mineral loss amounted to 6.4 percent. Long-term follow-up studies in hemiplegic patients may shed important light on the natural course of demineralization of paralyzed extremities and on the effect of spasticity and recovering neuromuscular function.

Metabolic Studies in Immobilization Osteoporosis

In the 1940s Albright and his associates[27] and Howard[28] reported the occurrence of hypercalciuria in patients who were immobilized for extended periods following lower-extremity fractures. The first systematic study on the metabolic effects of immobilization was done by Deitrick, Whedon, and Shorr.[29] Four healthy volunteers were immobilized in a plaster cast, which extended from the waist to the feet, and kept on bed rest for 6–7 weeks. The period of immobilization was preceded by a control period of 6–8 weeks and followed by a period or recovery lasting 4–6 weeks. The volunteers were on a rigidly controlled diet with a calcium intake just below 1 g/day. Urinary calcium began to rise on the second or third day of bed rest and reached its peak by the fourth to fifth week. The maximal 24-hr urinary excretion of calcium was more than double that of the control period in all four subjects. It remained on a plateau during the entire period of immobilization and gradually diminished during recovery. However, during the first 3 weeks of the recovery period, urinary calcium losses still exceeded control levels. The loss of calcium in the feces also rose during immobilization, reaching its peak during the latter weeks of bed rest. Total calcium losses, including the first 3 weeks of the recovery period, ranged from 8.95 to 23.9 g and averaged 14.1 g or 0.9 percent of the estimated total body calcium.

Urinary and fecal excretion of phosphorus was increased during bed rest, although fecal losses were small and variable. The urinary excretion showed two peaks, the first coinciding with the peak of nitrogen loss and the second peak (which occurred during the sixth to seventh week) appearing at the same time calcium excretion reached its maximum. Total phosphorus losses ranged from 5.1 to 11.6 g.

Later studies conducted with various experimental designs yielded similar results. Goldsmith,[30] working with healthy volunteers immobilized in a plaster cast for 40 days, noted a rapid rise of urinary calcium as soon as immobilization was instituted. The negative calcium balance (i.e., loss of calcium in urine and stool minus the dietary intake) averaged 152 mg/day. Donaldson and co-workers[31] confined three healthy male volunteers to 30–36 weeks of bed rest. Both urinary and fecal calcium losses reached their peaks during the seventh week, averaging 61 mg/day in excess of control level. The measured calcium loss during the entire period of bed rest was 4.2 percent of the estimated total body calcium with phosphorus excretion paralleling calcium loss.

Whedon, Shorr, and associates studied the calcium balance of patients paralyzed with acute anterior poliomyelitis.[32] Urinary calcium excretion reached its peak at the fifth week of illness. The average urinary excretion of calcium remained 250 mg/day above normal, on the average, for a period of 5½ months. The mean maximal negative calcium balance was greater than 500 mg/day. The calcium balance remained negative for an average of 7 months. It is of some interest that the calcium loss began to decrease before the patients began to ambulate. A positive balance was regained 1 month after ambulation had been resumed. The total calcium loss averaged 58 g or 4.2 percent of total body calcium. Radiographic evidence of bone demineralization first appeared in the pelvis and proximal femora when the calcium loss had reached 2 percent of total body calcium.

Rose reported urinary calcium measurements in 75 male and 64 female patients immobilized for extended periods because of lower extremity fractures.[33] Full balance studies were carried out only on a few patients. Females lost calcium during immobilization only slightly in excess of control values in contrast to the males, in whom the losses were significant. Urinary calcium excretion varied inversely with age in males but not in females, an observation not previously reported. The calcium loss through the feces was significantly increased. Rose attributed this to a failure of intestinal calcium absorption and concluded that the data supported a previously expressed theory that intestinal calcium absorption was regulated by endogenous factors, in response to the degree of saturation of the body with calcium. The rise of fecal calcium loss is, therefore, the result of osteoporosis due to disease or injury and not its cause. Rose's subjects lost 5–10 percent of their total body calcium; there is no evidence that this deficit is fully restored during recovery. These patients enter later adulthood with a decreased bone mass and, therefore, are subjected to the complication of osteoporosis earlier in life than others.

Millard, Nassim, and Woollen[34] reported significant hypercalciuria in five boys and seven girls who were immobilized for some months after a spinal fusion for scoliosis. Although considerable individual variations existed, the hypercalciuria began to decrease after 3 or 4 months in all cases. There was no difference between the sexes or with regard to the cause of the scoliosis.

An increase of urinary hydroxyproline and pyrophosphate have been reported by various investigators.[31] Chantraine found a good correlation between urinary hydroxyproline, calciuria, and loss of calcium from the total body pool in patients with paraplegia, quadriplegia, and cerebral trauma.[35] Claus-Walker *et al.* noted an increase of hydroxyproline excretion in quadriplegic patients which appeared within days after the injury and preceded the onset of hypercalcuria.[36] Urinary hydroxyproline decreased when the patients became engaged in rehabilitation exercises. At 18 months, urinary calcium, phosphorus, and hydroxyproline output were low. However, the urinary hydroxyproline again increased when patients were once more confined to bed at that point of time. The fact that the rise in hydroxyproline excretion precedes the hypercalciuria is consistent with the hypothesis that bone collagen resorption precedes demineralization. Klein and associates also reported that the hydroxyproline loss declined before the decrease of calciuria.[37]

Many investigators have supplemented metabolic balance studies with measurements of bone density. Mack and La Chance, utilizing a radiographic bone densitometry technique in healthy men on only 14 days of bed rest,[38] detected a decrease in the calcaneous bone mass which varied from 12 percent in individuals on a low calcium intake to 5 percent in those whose calcium intake was supplemented to 2 g a day. Donaldson and co-workers, who used gamma ray scanning densitometry in three men on prolonged bed rest, noted a decline of the calcaneous bone mass which began after 12 weeks.[31] One individual had lost 50 percent of bone mass by the 30th week; in the other two the loss was not quite as pronounced. All three individuals recovered full bone density with reambulation.

A recent report by Griffiths and co-workers deals with bone loss in the upper extremities of quadriplegic and paraplegic patients.[39] Scanning of the distal radius showed a selective loss of trabecular but not of cortical bone. The degree of demineralization was not related to the extent or duration of immobilization. Most remarkable is the observation that paraplegic patients with normal upper extremity function also showed a loss of trabecular bone in their distal radius, even though this was less marked than in quadriplegic patients. The authors emphasized that the discrepancy between cortical and trabecular bone loss in immobilization osteoporosis distinguishes this process from involutional osteoporosis in which bone loss involves both components. Why the upper extremities of paraplegic patients should be affected remains unexplained. Nikolic *et al.* performed radiographic studies of hands, feet, and femora of 100 paraplegic and quadriplegic patients.[40] They found that the cortical area was the best measure of bone strength. The cortical area was obtained from the equation $CA = D^2 - M^2$, where CA is the cortical area, D is the diameter of the diaphysis, and M is the diameter of the medullary cavity.

HYPERCALCEMIA IN IMMOBILIZATION

Hypercalcemia due to immobilization is a rare occurrence. It was first reported in 1941 by Albright.[27] His patient, a 14-year-old boy, developed bone atrophy, hypercalcemia, and renal failure during immobilization for a fractured femur. He underwent two neck explorations in a futile search for parathyroid tumors. Since Albright's original report, less than 50 cases have been reported in the literature. The subject has been reviewed by a number of authors.[41–45]

Almost all cases have occurred in adolescent young males who were physically active and in a phase of active bone growth just before they became immobilized. The only adults were patients with Paget's disease. It is obvious that a rapid bone turnover prior to injury is an important predisposing factor to the development of immobilization hypercalcemia. Hypercalcemia often developed after several weeks of immobilization. The patients complained of headaches, nausea, lethargy, constipation, and weakness. Emotional changes were often noted. Renal function studies showed a reduction of glomerular filtration rates. The ability to concentrate urine was decreased. In all patients the fractional excretion of calcium (the ratio of excreted to filtered calcium) was increased. Hyman[41] and Claus-Walker[44] also found the fractional excretion of phosphates to be increased. This suggests increased parathyroid activity, but hormone blood levels, whenever determined, were found to be in the low normal range. Hyman notes that immobilization hypercalcemia is commonly attended by a hypokalemic metabolic alkalosis. Steinberg et al. reported the case of a 15-year-old quadriplegic boy with immobilization hypercalcemia associated with adrenocortical insufficiency.[46] The hypercalcemia responded favorably to the administration of cortisone in replacement dosage.

Hypercalcemia of immobilization may not be as rare as the paucity of case reports suggests. Deitrick et al. [29] found an elevation of serum calcium above 12mg/100 ml in all of their immobilized volunteers. This occurred during the early phases of recovery. Heath and co-workers[47] reported an increase of ionized calcium in nine out of ten patients who were immobilized for the treatment of fractures. At the same time only three patients showed an increase of total serum calcium. In four healthy volunteers who were on complete bed rest for 12 days, the ionized serum calcium rose during or immediately after bed rest, while the total serum calcium remained normal. Urinary calcium excretion rose in all four subjects. The accumulated data suggest that milder forms of immobilization hypercalcemia may frequently remain undiscovered. The symptoms of nausea, headache, and weakness are not very specific and are not uncommon in injured and immobilized patients. Periodic serum calcium determinations in these patients may well uncover more cases with subtle and subclinical degrees of hypercalcemia.

Increasing the output of urine is important, both in preventing and treating immobilization hypercalciuria. Maynard reported on four adolescent male quadriplegics, two of whom became hypercalcemic while fluids were restricted as part of a program of intermittent catheterization.[48] Treatment therefore should include the promotion of diuresis by the administration of three to four liters of salt-containing intravenous fluids. Furosemide should be added to this regime. Serum potassium concentration must be monitored and supplementary potassium be given as needed. Oral phosphates promote a calcium diuresis and tend to lower serum calcium. They are often poorly tolerated, however. Calcitonin and prednisone are effective in lowering serum calcium. Anabolic steroids are also effective, probably by reducing bone resorption. Early mobilization, whenever possible, is still one of the more effective means of lowering elevated serum calcium levels, but exercises in bed fail to prevent or correct immobilization hypercalcemia.[45] The reduction of dietary calcium does not appear to be beneficial.

PREVENTION AND TREATMENT OF IMMOBILIZATION OSTEOPOROSIS

The interest in preventing or reducing loss of bone during immobilization has received a new impetus with the advent of space travel. Weightlessness produces physiologic effects very much akin to those of immobilization.

Whedon, Deitrick, and Shorr extended their original work on immobilized healthy men by investigating the effects of an oscillating bed.[49] Over a 2-min period, the bed rocked slowly from the horizontal to 20 degrees foot-down, and back to horizontal. This passive form of exercise was successful in reducing the urinary loss of calcium by one half. During the recovery phase, the calcium excretion returned to control levels more rapidly than it did following the fixed-bed immobilization. Issekutz[50] found that quiet standing for 3 hr per day induced a slow decline in the hypercalcuria of immobilized young men. However, exercise performed in the supine position for 4 hr/day or quiet sitting for 8 out of 24 hr failed to prevent the hypercalciuria. Issekutz concluded that pressure on the long bones is the physiologic stimulus required to maintain the balance between bone formation and resorption and to prevent osteoporosis. This stimulus cannot be replaced by the pulling force of intermittently exercising muscles. A daily 3-hr exposure to gravity appears to be the minimum required to prevent loss of bone substance.

On the other hand, Hantman[51] compressed the lower extremities and spine of healthy men on 19 weeks of bed rest with a force equal to 80 percent of body weight and failed to observe a reduction of the negative mineral balance. The compression force was applied in the recumbent position by a specially constructed apparatus 45 times/min for 4 hr/day. It is difficult to reconcile Hantman's negative observations with Issekutz' findings. It is possible that compression forces applied in the recumbent position are not equivalent to weight bearing or ambulation or that the muscular contractions in response to gravity play an important part in preventing bone demineralization. Supporting this assumption are earlier observations by the same group of investigators. Twelve weeks of bed rest in healthy men caused a considerable loss of mineral from the central calcaneus (measured by densitometry). While other forms of treatment were ineffective, ambulation after 30 weeks of recumbency quickly and totally restored the mineral content.[52] The recovery was complete within 10–20 weeks.

There is a good deal of conflicting information which indicates that demineralization is less responsive to weight bearing when the immobilization is due to paralysis, compared to healthy subjects on bed rest, or to patients immobilized for the treatment of fractures. In a long-term study of paraplegic patients, Abramson showed that 25 of 30 patients who did not walk or stand developed a marked osteoporosis of the lower extremities.[53] Only one of eight paraplegic patients who walked on braces and crutches for at least one hour a day, however, developed osteoporosis, and that to a mild degree. In a later survey of the literature, however, the same author casts considerable doubt on the effectiveness of weight bearing in the prevention of osteoporosis in patients with spinal-cord injury.[54] Rocking and oscillation, which had been so effective in reducing calcium losses in immobilized normal individuals, were quite ineffective in patients paralyzed by poliomyelitis.[55] In five paraplegic patients osteoporosis and hypercalcuria were not affected by the use of an oscillating bed or by standing on a tilt table. Plum and Dunning could demonstrate no fall in hypercalciuria in poliomyelitis patients who were exercised, mobilized in a wheelchair, rocked in bed, or who walked on crutches and braces.[56] The only patient who showed a significant fall in calcium output walked with canes, an activity which requires considerably more muscular activity. All of these observations suggest that in paralyzed patients the stimulus of weight bearing by itself is insufficient to prevent or retard osteoporosis and that muscular forces must also act on the bone. Abramson and Delagi have pointed out that these muscular forces are many times greater than the compression force of body weight.[54] Furthermore, muscles exert a variety of different forces upon bone—compressive, bending, shearing, and torsion—and each may have a specific effect in maintaining the balance between bone formation and resorption. As pointed out earlier in this chapter, compression and tension forces have different piezoelectric effects on bone.[14]

Claus-Walker[57] provided a somewhat different explanation for the failure of weight bearing to reduce or prevent bone loss in high-level spinal-cord lesions. She assumes the presence of baroceptors which transmit impulses to the central nervous system through neural pathways. In response, the central nervous system regulates calcium losses and sodium excretion mediated through the renin–angiotensin–aldosterone system. Obviously, these impulses cannot be transmitted through a transsected spinal cord.

The expansion of the extracellular fluid volume due to excessive sodium intake or excess adrenal cortical steroids produces hypercalciuria by reducing the absorption of calcium in the proximal tubules. Griffith reported that the combination of a low-sodium diet with a thiazide diuretic reduced calcium excretion by 53 percent in spinal-cord-injured patients.[58] Even better results were obtained in patients immobilized for the treatment of orthopedic conditions. These observations have been confirmed by Claus-Walker.[57] The hypercalciuria of paralyzed patients, which is greater than that in recumbency of normal individuals, was significantly reduced by sodium restriction, with or without the use of small amounts of thiazides. Larger doses of thiazides were ineffective in lowering the calcium loss, probably because they depleted the intracellular volume as well, thereby leaving the ratio of extracellular to intracellular fluid volume unchanged. Only measures which selectively reduce the extracellular fluid compartment will be effective in diminishing calcium losses through excessive renal excretion. Sodium restriction with or without the use of small doses of diuretics may, therefore, be an effective therapeutic method of preventing excessive calcium losses during immobilization.

Goldsmith and co-workers reported that phosphate supplements decrease the urinary excretion of calcium during recumbency.[30] Six healthy men were immobilized in plaster casts for 40 days. Supplements of 1–2 g of phosphate daily decreased the urinary excretion of calcium and to a lesser extent reduced the negative calcium balance. This effect was present in individuals who received the supplements from the start of immobilization. In other subjects hypercalciuria and crystalluria were reversed by phosphate supplementation after about 40 days of immobilization. Hulley et al.[52] studied five healthy young men on 24–30 weeks of complete bed rest. Potassium phosphate supplements prevented the hypercalciuria of bed rest but increased fecal calcium losses. During the first 12 weeks the calcium balance was slightly less negative. This effect was not apparent during the second 12 weeks. The mineral losses from the central calcaneus were not affected. Hydroxyproline excretion and serum alkaline phosphatase levels were not changed by phosphate supplementation. The authors conclude that phosphate supplementation, while reducing urinary calcium excretion, does not prevent bone loss during immobilization and by itself is not an effective way of averting or treating disuse osteoporosis. Hantman and co-workers[51] confined six healthy young men to 19 weeks of complete bed rest. An increase of calcium intake to approximately 2 g/day and of phosphorus intake to about 3 g/day significantly lowered the negative calcium balance, compared to control subjects. The increase of hydroxyproline excretion of recumbency was significantly lowered by this regime. There was no effect on the serum alkaline phosphatase levels or on the demineralization of the central calcaneus. These data indicate that a combined phosphate and calcium supplementation is effective in diminishing bone resorption during immobilization while phosphate supplements alone appear to be ineffective. However, the clinical and therapeutic implications of these observations, when applied to long-term immobilization and paralysis, remain uncertain.

Calcitonin appeared to have promise in the treatment of osteoporosis because it inhibits bone resorption upon short-term administration. The results have been disappointing. In a preliminary study, Wynston and Perkins could demonstrate that the decalcification of legs of rats immobilized by plaster casts could be prevented by porcine calcitonin.[59] Chiroff and Jowsey, however, reported that calcitonin given in sufficient dosage to lower serum calcium failed to prevent osteoporosis in the immobilized legs of dogs.[60] They surmised that the long-term administration of calcitonin stimulated an excessive production of parathyroid hormone which cancelled out whatever bone mass sparing effect the calcitonin might have. Braddom found calcitonin ineffective in preventing osteoporosis in paraplegic rats.[61]

Hantman and co-workers gave 100 MRC units of synthetic salmon calcitonin to four of six young men confined to bed rest, either alone or in combination with calcium and phosphorus supplements and intermittent longitudinal bone compression.[51] Calcitonin, unless combined with calcium and phosphorus supplements, failed to prevent the development of a negative calcium balance. One subject actually showed rises of urinary calcium and hydroxyproline in excess to those observed during control periods. One subject also showed a significant loss of mineral from the calcaneus. The increased excretion of calcium in the urine may be due to inhibition of tubular reabsorption which had been previously described. The authors concluded that calcitonin given in a dosage effective in the treatment of Paget's disease did not by itself prevent disuse osteoporosis and did not add to the salutary effect of calcium and phosphate supplements. They, too, suggested that the failure may be due to stimulation of parathyroid hormone production mediated by hypocalcemia even though they were unable to demonstrate significant changes in the blood levels of serum calcium, ionized calcium, or parathyroid hormone.

The effect of diphosphanates (well-established inhibitors of bone resorption) was investigated by Lockwood and associates.[62] Four healthy young men were confined to 20 weeks of bed rest. The administration of diphosphanates was begun 3 days before the commencement of immobilization. Two subjects received 5 mg/kg/day of disodium etidronate and two subjects received 20 mg/kg/day. The data were compared to controls obtained from a previous study in which immobilized individuals had remained untreated.

The two subjects who received the higher dosage of disodium etidronate showed an immediate sharp rise of urinary and fecal calcium excretion. In contrast to the controls, the urinary hydroxyproline excretion decreased during bed rest. Serum phosphorus levels rose while the serum alkaline phosphatase activity declined. Bone accretion and resorption rates fell progressively to levels 50 percent below baseline by the end of bed rest. After 12 weeks of bed rest, calcium and phosphorus balance shifted toward positive, but the loss of mineral from the calcaneus remained unaffected. The subjects on the low-dosage regimen showed only minor drug effects. The increase of bone accretion, usually seen in the early phase of immobilization, was prevented, and the urinary hydroxyproline excretion was accentuated.

Previous work had suggested that there may be an optimal dosage of diphosphonate which inhibits bone resorption without decreasing bone accretion.[63] The authors conclude from their observations that such an optimal dosage may not exist. The lower dosage, which was relatively ineffective, suppressed accretion more than resorption, while the higher dosage suppressed both components. Although it is possible, that continued administration of diphosphonates in a dose of 20 mg/kg/day beyond 20 weeks might lower the extent of mineral loss from bone, there is presently no evidence to support this assumption. Moreover, this form of therapy appears contraindicated, since high-dose diphosphonate treatment does produce osteomalacia and may increase the incidence of fractures.[64]

Early observers reported on the therapeutic value of anabolic hormones. Whedon and Shorr found that testosterone decreased the mineral loss in poliomyelitis patients.[65] The addition of estradiol offered a clear advantage and also reduced the tendency to urinary calculus formation by increasing the renal excretion of citric acid. Plum and Dunning also noted that anabolic steroids improved the calcium balance by reducing the urinary elimination of calcium.[66] Heaney reported that anabolic steroids improved the calcium balance both in the acute and chronic phases of immobilization osteoporosis.[21] In the acute phase this effect was entirely due to a reduction of bone resorption. Bone formation was not increased.

No recent evidence has been presented that gonadal hormones or their anabolic derivatives are beneficial in the management of immobilization osteoporosis. In summary, immobilization osteoporosis is most effectively managed by mobilization of the patient whenever possible. A good deal of evidence suggests that mobilization should include weight bearing and muscular activity for maximal effectiveness. The hypercalciuria of immobilized patients can be effectively reduced by thiazide medication, and the complications of increased urinary calcium can be minimized by hydration. Supplementary forms of therapy such as dietary calcium and phosphorus, calcitonin, and diphosphonates have proved less than adequate in reversing the tendency toward osteoporosis and calciuria.

REFERENCES

1. Von Volkmann, R. *Handbuch der allgemeinen und speziellen Chirurgie*, p. 282, 1882.
2. Legg, A. The cause of atrophy in joint disease. *Am. J. Orthop. Surg.* 6:84, 1908.
3. Willert, H. G. Immobilisationsosteoporose. Langenbecks. *Arch. Klin. Chir.* 315:258, 1966.
4. Jenkins, D. P. and Cochran, T. H. The dramatic effect of disuse of an extremity. *Clin. Orthop.* 64:128, 1969.
5. Haike, H. J., Heymann, P., and Wagner, K. Experimentelle Untersuchungen ueber den Einfluss der Immobilisation auf die Knochenfestigkeit und Knochenelastizitaet sowie ueber die Regenerationsfaehigkeit derselben bei der Remobilisation. *Z. Orthop.* 102:200, 1966–1967.
6. Whedon, G. D. Osteoporosis: Atrophy of disuse. In: *Bone as a Tissue* (K. Rodahl, ed.). New York, 1960. McGraw-Hill Co.
7. Geiser, M., and Trueta, J. Muscle action, bone rarification and bone formation. *J. Bone Jt. Surg.* 40B:282, 1958.
8. Hulth, A., and Olerud, S. Disease of extremities. II. A microangiographic study in the rabbit, *Acta Chir. Scand.* 120:388, 1961.

9. Sundén, G. Some aspects of longitudinal bone growth. An experimental study in the rabbit. *Acta Orthop. Scand.*, Suppl. 103, 1967.
10. Hardt, A. B. Early metabolic responses of bone to immobilization. *J. Bone Jt. Surg.* **54A**:119, 1972.
11. Little, K., and De Valderrama, J. F. Some mechanisms involved in the osteoporotic process. *Gerontologia* **14**:109, 1968.
12. Trueta, J. Der Einfluss des Muskels auf den Blutstrom in den langen Roehrenknochen. *Z. Orthop.* **99**:11, 1964/1965.
13. De Valderrama, J. F., and Trueta, J. The effect of muscle action on the intraosseous circulation. *J. Pathol. Bacteriol.* **89**:179, 1965.
14. Harris, W. H., and Heaney, R. P. Skeletal renewal and metabolic bone disease. *N. Engl. J. Med.* **280**:193, 253, 303, 1969.
15. Doyle, F., Brown, J., and LaChance, C. *Lancet* **1**:391, 1970.
16. Landry, M., and Fleisch, H. The influence of immobilization on bone formation as evaluated by osseous incorporation of tetracyclines. *J. Bone Jt. Surg.* **46B**:764, 1964.
17. Pennock, J. M., Kalu, D. N., Clark, M. B., Foster, G. V., and Doyle, F. H. Hypoplasia of bone induced by immobilization. *Br. J. Radiol.* **45**:641, 1972.
18. Mattson, S. The reversibility of disuse osteoporosis. *Acta Orthop. Scand.*, Suppl. 144, 1972.
19. Uhthoff, H. K. and Jaworski, Z. F. G. Bone loss in response to long-term immobilization. *J. Bone Jt. Surg.* **60B**:420, 1978.
20. Burkhart, J. M., and Jowsey, J. Parathyroid and thyroid hormones in the development of disuse osteoporosis. *Endocrinology* **81**:1053, 1967.
21. Heaney, R. P. Radiocalcium metabolism in disuse osteoporosis in man. *Am. J. Med.* **33**:188, 1962.
22. Minaire, P., Meunier, P., Edouard, C., Bernard, J., Courpron, P., and Bourret, J. Quantitative histological data on disuse osteoporosis. *Calcif. Tissue Res.* **17**:57, 1974.
23. Nilsson, E. R. Post-traumatic osteopenia. *Acta Orthop. Scand.*, Suppl. 91, 1966.
24. Hodkinson, H. M., and Brain, A. T. Unilateral osteoporosis in long-standing hemiplegia in the elderly. *J. Am. Geriatr. Soc.* **15**:59, 1967.
25. Panin, N., Gorday, W. J., and Paul, B. J. Osteoporosis in hemiplegia. *Stroke* **2**:41, 1971.
26. Naftchi, N. E., Viau, A., Marshall, C. H., Davis, W. S., and Lowman, E. W. Bone mineralization in the distal forearm of hemiplegic patients. *Arch. Phys. Med. Rehab.* **56**:487, 1975.
27. Albright, F., Burnett, C. H., Cope, O., and Parson, W. Acute atrophy of bone (osteoporosis) simulating hyperparathyroidism. *J. Clin. Endocrinol.* **1**:711, 1941.
28. Howard, J. E., Parson, W., and Bigham, R. S., Jr. Studies on patients

convalescent from fracture. III. The urinary excretion of calcium and phosphorus. *Bull. Johns Hopkins Hosp.* **77**:291, 1945.

29. Deitrick, J. E., Whedon, G. D., and Shorr, E. Effects of immobilization upon various metabolic and physiologic functions of normal men. *Am. J. Med.* **4**:3, 1948.
30. Goldsmith, R. S., Killian, P., Ingbar, S. H., and Bass, D. E. Effect of phosphate supplementation during immobilization of normal men. *Metabolism* **18**:349, 1969.
31. Donaldson, C. L., Hulley, S. B., Vogel, J. M., Hattner, R. S., Bayers, J. H., and McMillan, D. E. Effect of prolonged bedrest on bone mineral. *Metabolism* **19**:1071, 1970.
32. Whedon, G. D., Shorr, E., Toscani, V., and Stevens, E. Metabolic studies in paralytic anterior poliomyelitis. II. Alteration in calcium and phosphorus metabolism. *J. Clin. Invest.* **36**:966, 1957.
33. Rose, G. A. Immobilization osteoporosis. Study of the extent, severity, and treatment with bendrofluazide. *Br. J. Surg.* **53**:769, 1966.
34. Millard, F. J. C., Nassim, J. R., and Woollen, J. W. Urinary calcium excretion after immobilization and spinal fusion in adolescents. *Arch. Dis. Child.* **45**:399, 1970.
35. Chantraine, A. Clinical investigation of bone metabolism in spinal cord lesions. *Paraplegia* **8**:253, 1970/1971.
36. Claus-Walker, J., Spencer, W. A., Carter, R. E., Halstead, L. S., Meier, R. H. III, and Campos, R. J. Bone metabolism in quadriplegia: Dissociation between calciuria and hydroxyprolinuria. *Arch. Phys. Med. Rehab.* **56**:327, 1975.
37. Klein, L., Van Den Noort, S., and DeJak, J. J. Sequential studies of urinary hydroxyproline and serum alkaline phosphatase in acute paraplegia. *Med. Serv. J. Can.* **22**:524, 1966.
38. Mack, P. B., and La Chance, P. L. Effects of recumbency and space flight on bone density. *Am. J. Clin. Nutr.* **20**:1194, 1967.
39. Griffiths, H. J., Bushueff, B., and Zimmerman, R. E. Investigation of the loss of bone mineral in patients with spinal cord injury. *Paraplegia* **14**:207, 1976.
40. Nikolic, V., Vladovic, P., Sajko, D., Zimmermann, B., Hudec, M., Vladovic, A., Hancevic, J., and Mijatovic, Z. Bone mass and safety factor of bone strength in lower extremities of patients with paraplegia. *Calcif. Tissue Res.* **22**:(Suppl) 303, 1977.
41. Hyman, L. R., Boner, G., Thomas, J. C., and Segar, W. E., Immobilization hypercalcemia. *Am. J. Dis. Child.* **124**:723, 1972.
42. Lawrence, G. D., Loeffler, R. G., Martin, L. G., and Connor, T. B. Immobilization hypercalcemia. *J. Bone Jt. Surg.* **55A**:87, 1973.
43. Wolf, A. W., Chuinard, R. G., Riggins, R. S., Walter, R. M., and Depner, T. Immobilization hypercalcemia. *Clin. Orthop.* **118**:124, 1976.

44. Claus-Walker, J., Carter, R. E., Campos, R. J., and Spencer, W. A. Hypercalcemia in early traumatic quadriplegia. *J. Chron. Dis.* **28**:81, 1975.

45. Rosen, J. F., Wolin, D. A., and Finberg, L. Immobilization hypercalcemia after single limb fracture in children and adolescents. *Am. J. Dis. Child.* **132**:560, 1978.

46. Steinberg, F. U., Birge, S. J., and Cooke, N. E. Hypercalcemia in adolescent tetraplegic patients: Case report and review. *Paraplegia* **16**:60, 1978.

47. Heath, H., III, Earll, J. M., Schaaf, M., Piechocki, J. T., and Ting-Kai Li. Serum ionized calcium during bedrest in fracture patients and normal men. *Metabolism* **21**:633, 1972.

48. Maynard, F. M., and Imai, K. Immobilization hypercalcemia in spinal cord injury. *Arch. Phys. Med. Rehab.* **58**:16, 1977.

49. Whedon, G. D., Deitrick, J. E., and Shorr, E. Modification of the effect of immobilization upon metabolic and physiologic functions of normal men by the use of an oscillating bed. *Am. J. Med.* **6**:684, 1949.

50. Issekutz, B. Jr., Blizzard, J. J., Birkhead, N. C., and Rodahl, K. Effect of prolonged bed rest on urinary calcium output. *J. Appl. Physiol.* **21**:1013, 1966.

51. Hantman, D. A., Vogel, J. M., Donaldson, C. L., Friedman, R., Goldsmith, R. S., and Hulley, S. B. Attempts to prevent disuse osteoporosis by treatment with calcitonin, longitudinal compression and supplementary calcium and phosphate. *J. Clin. Endocrinol. Metab.* **36**:845, 1973.

52. Hulley, S. B., Vogel, J. M., Donaldson, C. L., Bayers, J. H., Friedman, R. J., and Rosen, S. N. The effect of supplemental oral phosphate on the bone mineral changes during prolonged bed rest. *J. Clin. Invest.* **50**:2506, 1971.

53. Abramson, A. S. Bone disturbances in injuries to the spinal cord and cauda equina (paraplegia). Their prevention by ambulation. *J. Bone Jt. Surg.* **30A**:982, 1948.

54. Abramson, A. S. and Delagi, E. F. Influence of weight-bearing and muscle contraction on disuse osteoporosis. *Arch. Phys. Med. Rehab.* **42**:147, 1961.

55. Wyse, D. M., and Pattee, C. J. Effect of the oscillating bed and tilt table on calcium, phosphorus and nitrogen metabolism in paraplegia. *Am. J. Med.* **17**:645, 1954.

56. Plum, F., and Dunning, M. F. The effect of therapeutic mobilization on hypercalcuria following acute poliomyelitis. *Arch. Int. Med.* **101**:528, 1958.

57. Claus-Walker, J., Campos, R. J., Carter, R. E., Vallbona, C., and

Lipscomb, H. S. Calcium excretion in quadriplegia. *Arch. Phys. Med. Rehab.* **53**:14, 1972.

58. Griffith, D. P. Immobilization hypercalciuria: Treatment and possible pathophysiologic mechanism. *Aerosp. Med.* **42**:1322, 1971.

59. Wynston, L. K., and Perkins, D. L. Effectiveness of thyrocalcitonin in maintaining bone strength *in vivo* under decalcifying conditions. *Aerosp. Med.* **39**:966, 1968.

60. Chiroff, R. T., and Jowsey, J. The effect of calcitonin on immobilization osteopenia. *J. Bone Jt. Surg.* **52A**:1138, 1970.

61. Braddom, R. L., Erickson, R., and Johnson, E. W. Ineffectiveness of calcitonin on osteoporosis in paraplegic rats. *Arch. Phys. Med. Rehab.* **54**:170, 1973.

62. Lockwood, D. R., Vogel, J. M., Schneider, V. S., and Hulley, S. B. Effect of the diphosphanate EHDP on bone mineral metabolism during prolonged bedrest. *J. Clin. Endocrinol. Metab.* **41**:533, 1975.

63. King, W. R., Francis, M. D., and Michael, W. R. Effect of Disodium ethane-1-hydroxy-1-diphosphanate on bone formation. *Clin. Orthop.* **78**:251, 1971.

64. Canfield, R., Rosner, W., Skinner, J., McWorther, J., Resnick, F., Feldman, F., Kammerman, S., Ryan, K., Kunigonis, M., and Bohne, W. Diphosphonate therapy of Paget's disease of bone. *J. Clin. Endocrinol. Metab.* **44**:96, 1977.

65. Whedon, G. D., and Shorr, E. Metabolic studies in paralytic acute anterior poliomyelitis. IV. Effects of testosterone proprionate and estradiol benzoate on calcium, phosphorus, nitrogen and creatine metabolism, *J. Clin. Invest.* **36**:995, 1957.

66. Plum, F., and Dunning, M. F. Amelioration of hypercalcuria following poliomyelitis by 17-ethyl-19-nortesterone (Nilevar). *J. Clin. Endocrinol.* **18**:860, 1958.

CHAPTER 4

Immobilization and Skeletal Muscles

Skeletal muscle and immobilization are linked in a dual causal relationship. Muscle paralysis is an obvious cause of immobilization. On the other hand, when muscles are immobilized by extraneous forces they undergo changes which may permanently affect their structure and function.

Physiology of Muscle

Skeletal muscle makes up 40 percent of the body mass. Oxygen consumption and blood flow vary considerably with the degree of activity. A contracting muscle consumes 25–30 times more oxygen than it does at rest. The blood flow through an exercising muscle reaches 15–20 times the resting value. It is obvious that the immobilization of a major portion of the muscle mass has a profound effect on the body metabolism as a whole, as well as on circulation and respiration.

The contractile unit of skeletal muscle is the myofibril, which is composed of thick myosin and thin actin filaments. The immediate source of energy for muscle contraction is ATP (adenosine triphosphate), which breaks down into ADP (adenosine diphosphate) and phosphate. This reaction releases 7.6 kCal of energy per mole of ATP. Less than one

65

second of muscular activity depletes the ATP stores. In order for muscular contractions to continue, ATP must be reconstituted from ADP and phosphates, with energy being supplied from various backup systems. The immediate energy source for the replenishing ATP is provided by the breakdown of creatine phosphate. However, this source is also depleted within a few seconds of intense muscular activity. Tertiary energy supplies are provided by the metabolism of carbohydrates and free fatty acids. This source is available to the contracting muscle for a long period of time, provided that the circulation continues to supply the oxygen that is needed to metabolize glucose and fatty acids to their metabolic end points. If the oxygen delivery lags, anaerobic processes leading to the production of lactic acid are called into play. The energy-producing metabolic processes take place in the mitochondria, which are bacteria-sized bodies found in juxtaposition to the myosin and actin filaments within the myofibrils.[1,2]

The functional entity of the skeletal muscle is the motor unit, consisting of an anterior horn cell from which an alpha nerve fiber originates. It branches into small motor fibers which terminate at the myoneural junctions and carry impulses to the muscle fibers. The ratio of muscle fibers per anterior horn cell is extremely variable. Muscles which perform finely coordinated movements, such as the eye muscles, carry a much smaller number of muscle fibers in each motor unit than do muscles that function by gross forceful contractions.

Different motor units vary in the force that the contracting muscle fibers generate. The larger the motor unit the greater is the force of contraction. In the same muscle the larger motor units can be as much as 50 times as strong as the smallest units. The force with which a muscle as a whole contracts depends on the number and size of motor units that are recruited and on their rate of firing. The small motor units are recruited first. As the contraction becomes increasingly forceful, larger and larger motor units are activated. Each individual unit when first recruited will fire at a minimum rate of 5 discharges/sec. At this slow rate, the muscle fibers relax completely between twitches. At rates from 10/sec upward the muscle fibers will have not yet returned to their resting length when the next impulse arrives. Therefore, the second contraction is superimposed on the one preceding it, leading to a summation of twitches. At firing rates of 40/sec and above, the individual twitches are fused into a smooth tetanic contraction. In human muscle a firing rate of 50/sec seems to constitute the upper limit. Different motor units fire in asynchrony to each other. While one motor unit relaxes another begins to contract. This asynchrony provides for smooth contractions, even at rates of firing that are not frequent enough to cause tetanization. The force with which a muscle contracts is under the volitional control of the central nervous system. This control determines simultaneously how many motor units are to be recruited and the rates at which they fire. Normal muscle contractions are tetanic because of the fusion of individual twitches.

Muscle fibers are distinguished by their contractile characteristics. Fast-twitch Type II fibers reach their peak tensions two to four times as rapidly as the slow-twitch Type I fibers. Their relaxation time is equally as rapid. They fatigue more readily than slow-twitch fibers. Fast-twitch fibers have smaller and fewer mitochondria. They are rich in phosphorylase, and they are glycolytic, that is they use glucose in preference to fatty acids for energy production. Slow-twitch Type I fibers have a high oxidative capacity and predominantly use fatty acids as fuel. They have a red color due to their greater blood supply and a higher myoglobin content. An individual motor unit is solely composed of either Type I or Type II fibers. In some animals muscles are either red or white, that is they are entirely composed of Type I or Type II fibers. Human muscles contain both fast-twitch or slow-twitch fibers, with one type predominating over the other, depending on the function of the muscle. Cross innervation experiments, transposing nerves from slow-twitch to fast-twitch muscles or vice versa alter the contractile characteristics of the muscle and convert them from one type to the other.[3] Recent experiments have shown that long-term electrical stimulation can convert fast-twitch to slow-twitch motor units.[4]

Fast-twitch and slow-twitch muscles have different functions. Antigravity muscles which are concerned with maintaining posture consist mostly of slow-twitch fibers. Thus the erector muscles of the spine or the soleus are of the slow-twitch variety. They can hold a tonic contraction of low but steady intensity for long periods of time. Muscles which carry predominantly fast-twitch fibers are best suited for rapid short-term phasic movements.

The strength of a muscle, that is the maximal force that it can develop varies directly with its cross section. Muscles contract against external loads. A muscle shortens in a concentric contraction if it is strong enough to overcome the load resistance. If muscle strength and load are equal, the contraction is isometric, that is, the muscle contracts without changing its length. If a muscle resists and yet is overpowered by an extraneous stretching force, it performs an eccentric contraction. In this case, while the myofibrils contract the muscle lengthens in an effort to overcome the extraneous stretching force. The active tension which an isolated muscle can generate by an isometric contraction depends upon its

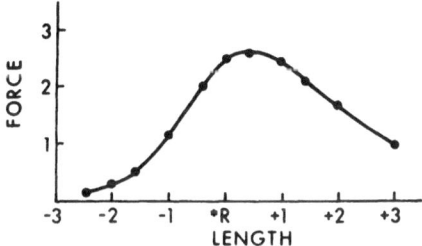

FIGURE 3. Relationship of tension to length for an isolated muscle preparation (deducting the elastic force of the stretched muscle). Modified from Howard G. Knuttgen, *Neuromuscular Mechanisms for Therapeutic and Conditioning Exercise*, University Park Press, 1976, with permission of the author and publisher.

length. This has been demonstrated in experiments in which the same maximal tetanizing current was applied to a muscle, and the various initial lengths were plotted against the force of the contraction. The maximal tension is generated when the muscle is slightly stretched past resting length. As the muscle is stretched further, the tension diminishes (provided that the purely passive elastic resistance against stretch is subtracted from the total measured tension). On the other side to the peak, as the muscle shortens, the tension also decreases. When an active muscle is shortened to more than 60 percent of its resting length, the tension becomes zero. Muscles, therefore, contract most efficiently and forcefully when they are on slight stretch at the beginning of the contraction (Figure 3).

The velocity of contraction also affects the force of a muscular contraction. In concentric shortening contractions, the force diminishes with increasing velocities. For all velocities the force of concentric contractions is less than the one developed by an isometric contraction. For lengthening contractions, however, the muscle force rises with the velocity up to a maximum at which the curve levels out (Figure 4).

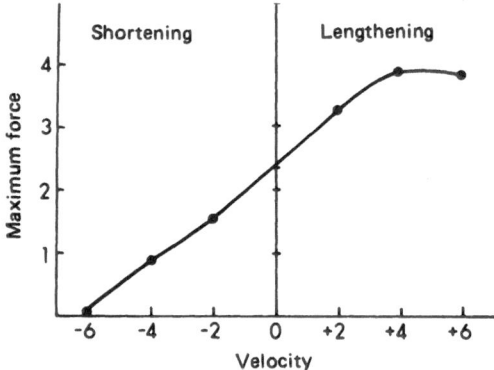

FIGURE 4. Relationship of force to velocity of contraction for an isolated muscle preparation under maximal electrical stimulation. Modified from Howard G. Knuttgen, *Neuromuscular Mechanisms for Therapeutic and Conditioning Exercise,* University Park Press, 1976, with permission of the author and publisher.

The foregoing facts, as well as other clinical and experimental observations, allow the following conclusions.

• Strength is the maximal force which a muscle can develop. It is related to the cross section of the muscle.

• Endurance is the ability of a muscle to perform work of less than maximal intensity for prolonged periods of time. In everyday life endurance is more important than maximal strength. We rarely need all of the force which a muscle can muster. Most of our everyday activities, however, are contingent upon endurance.

• Continuing muscular activity depends upon a steady supply of fuel and oxygen. Carbohydrate and fatty acids, needed to restore the high energy phosphate compounds, are available in sufficient quantities, and the supply lasts for an adequate period of time. Oxygen, however, cannot be stored. Muscular activity can continue only as long as respiration and circulation can deliver oxygen to the working muscles. Anaerobic metabolic processes can be utilized for only brief periods of intense activity. The ensuing lactic acid oxygen debt needs to be paid off promptly. Lower level muscular activities for which oxygen delivery can keep up with demands can be maintained indefinitely.

• Muscles contract most forcefully when they are on slight stretch at the beginning of the contraction. During walking, for instance, the hip flexors are at an advantage if they are first stretched by hip extension. Initial stretch is particularly advantageous to those muscles which cross two joints. For example, the hamstrings act as hip extensors and knee flexors. The knee flexor function is more forceful when the hamstrings are under stretch by simultaneous hip flexion.

Within the intact musculoskeletal system, however, initial muscle length is not the only factor determining the torque with which one bone is moved against another. The laws of leverage provide mechanical advantages at certain joint angles, depending upon the relationship of the length of the force arm to the length of the load arm.[5]* In certain instances these mechanical advantages may outweigh the physiologic benefit of the initial stretch. For example, the chief flexors of the elbow, the biceps and the brachialis, have their greatest torque not at elbow extension when they are at full stretch but at 90 degrees; at that angle leverage makes for an optimum mechanical advantage. When weights are lifted through the full range of a joint, the mechanical advantage varies at different points of the arc of motion. Where the muscle works at a mechanical advantage, less force needs to be expended. More force needs to be generated in those sectors of the arc where the muscle works at a mechanical disadvantage. The total amount of weight that can be lifted

*Mechanical advantage = Force arm/load arm.

depends upon the force that a muscle can develop at that point of the arc where it operates under the greatest mechanical disadvantage. The weakest link determines the strength of a chain.

• The muscle force decreases with the velocity of contraction. In weight lifting the motion automatically accelerates in those sectors of the arc where mechanical advantages ease the load on the muscle. Both effort and training effect, therefore, become uneven. Isokinetic exercises hold the exercising muscles to a constant velocity and do not permit a relaxation of effort at the easy sectors of the arc.[6]

MUSCLE TESTING

Our knowledge of the specific function of individual muscles has been derived from studying their anatomic relationship to bones and joints, the study of cadavers and the observation of movements of normal individuals and of patients with paralyses. Duchenne developed a system of kinesiology by observing the contractions of electrically stimulated muscles.[7] During the last few decades electromyographic methods have been widely used to elucidate the function of individual muscles.[8,9]

One or several muscles may be the prime movers in specific joint movements. To perform this particular movement is their major function. Muscles that perform the opposite movement are called antagonists. Examples are wrist flexors and wrist extensors, hip abductors and adductors, etc. Synergists are muscles which assist with a specific movement, even though this is not their primary function. For instance, the extensor carpi radialis is primarily an extensor of the wrist but it also aids synergistically with elbow flexion. The extensor of the big toe is a synergist to the dorsi-flexor (the anterior tibialis) of the ankle. Another group of muscles serves as stabilizer of one portion of the skeleton against which another portion is moved. Prime examples are the muscles which firmly hold the shoulder girdle against the chest wall, the rhomboids, trapezius, pectoralis minor, etc. The shoulder girdle has no bony or firm ligamentous attachment to the thorax. The humerus cannot be forcefully abducted, flexed, or rotated unless the scapula against which the humerus is to move is stabilized by muscle action. In-ability to produce a motion in the shoulder joint may, there-fore, result from weakness of, e.g., the deltoid, which is a prime mover, or from weakness of the stabilizers. The wrist extensors act as stabilizers for finger movements.

A system of muscle testing was first described by Dr. Robert W. Lovett, an orthopedic surgeon in Boston. His chief objective was the evaluation of patients with poliomyelitis. Since this disease attacks individual muscles, regardless of their nerve supply or segmental spinal cord innervation, it was important to develop tests that could measure the func-tion of each individual muscle. Lovett's system has been modified but the principle of his methodology has remained intact. Muscles are tested for their ability to overcome resis-tance or gravity. Each muscle is tested for its primary func-tion. The limb is positioned in such a way that only that muscle can perform the test movement and that the partici-pation of synergists is excluded.

Various grading systems have been designed. The sys-tem now most commonly used has been developed by the National Foundation for Infantile Paralysis. It uses six major grades:

1. Normal—Complete range of motion against gravity with full resistance.

2. Good—Complete range of motion against gravity with some resistance.
3. Fair—Complete range of motion against gravity (without resistance).
4. Poor—Complete range of motion with gravity eliminated.
5. Trace—Palpable contraction but no joint motion.
6. Zero—No demonstrable contraction.

There are intermediate grades, e.g., "Fair plus" or "Fair minus." "Fair minus" indicates to many observers that a joint can be moved against gravity but not through full range. Testing procedures for individual muscles are described in two monographs which serve as guides to physicians and physical therapists. [10,11]

Neurologists prefer to grade muscle from 0 to 5, with 5 signifying normal strength. Unfortunately, systems are also in use in which 0 means normal strength, and 5 means total paralysis.

Manual muscle testing has its limitations. The gauging of grades above the "fair" level becomes subject to considerable observer bias. Two examiners, or the same examiner on different days, may have difficulties in deciding if a grade is "normal" or "good." The use of gravity as an index of muscle strength is not possible for all muscles. For instance, there is no way of determining if the supinators or pronators of the forearm can perform their movements against the pull of gravity. Some muscles can be best tested in a functional position. The gastrocnemius–soleus group is best tested by having the individual rise on tiptoes. The ability to stand on tiptoe with the knee flexed tests the soleus specifically since gastrocnemius function is eliminated in this position. The ability to stand on one leg is a good test for the hip abductors, specifically the gluteus medius. With the foot firmly on the ground the hip abductors hold the center of gravity over the supporting leg.

The system of manual muscle testing was designed for poliomyelitis, a condition in which it is important to assess the strength of each muscle individually. This is not necessary for the evaluation of many neurologic conditions in which it may be just as informative to gauge the strength of movements rather than of single muscles. Into how much detail one wishes to go depends upon the tentative diagnosis. Muscles that perform the same function may have different nerve supplies and may arise from different spinal levels. In this case it may be necessary to test individual muscles separately. In many situations, however, a screening examination of total movements will suffice. A complete manual muscle test is very time-consuming. It will tire the patient and take up personnel time which may be used to advantage for other activities.

The validity of the conventional muscle tests for upper motor lesions has been questioned. In patients with cerebral involvement, the strength of a movement may depend upon the position of the limb, the posture of the head and neck, etc. In some instances gravity may have a facilitating effect so that a movement is performed better against gravity than with gravity eliminated. In the evaluation of patients with strokes or head injuries muscle examination must be performed with this consideration in mind.

MUSCLE PARALYSIS AS A CAUSE OF IMMOBILIZATION

A total body paralysis of all of the skeletal muscles of trunk and extremities is rare. It may occur in high-level cervical-cord lesions or in degenerative neurologic disorders such as advanced multiple sclerosis. When only some muscles are paralyzed prime movers may be overpowered by their antagonists. It is the role of the Rehabilitation Medicine staff to train the synergists to perform new functions if the prime movers cannot be restored and to prevent the adverse effect that the uninhibited antagonists may have on the total movement pattern.

Depending on the cause, the paralysis may be flaccid or spastic. Flaccid muscles are encountered in lesions which affect the lower motor neurons and in primary muscle diseases. Moderate spasticity may be a mechanical advantage. Patients become very skillful in initiating spastic muscular responses and utilizing them to facilitate motions. Paraplegic patients can bear their weight for brief moments on spastically extended limbs, long enough to help them transfer from one place to the other. Turning over in bed is easier when the lower extremity muscles have some tone. When they are totally flaccid they are dead weight, and the patient who wishes to turn in bed may have to reposition them manually or need the assistance of another person. Excessive spasticity is destructive to body movements. Unopposed spastic muscles will overpower their weak antagonists causing shortening and joint contractures. Forceful involuntary spastic contractions may throw patients out of the wheelchair or bed. When spasticity becomes a detriment to body position or locomotion it will have to be treated, either by medication or destructive surgical procedures. Rhizotomies or alcohol instillation into the spinal canal permanently convert spasticity to flaccidity. Because of the mechanical disadvantages engendered by flaccidity the indications for such destructive procedures have to be weighed carefully. Intrathecal phenol instillation selectively destroys the small diameter gamma fibers and leaves a portion of the alpha fibers intact. This procedure therefore can relieve spasticity without rendering the muscles totally flaccid. The effect, however, may be short-lived and the procedure may have to be repeated. [12]

The Effect of Denervation and Immobilization on Muscle

If the neural elements of a motor unit, that is, the anterior horn cell or the nerve fibers, are destroyed, the muscle fibers degenerate in a characteristic fashion. They atrophy at an even rate and eventually their volume is only 5 to 10 percent of normal, while the connective tissue and blood vessel bulk is preserved. The sarcolemmal nuclei appear increased in number and are located centrally within the atrophic fiber. If reinnervation does not occur within a given period of time—and this may vary from several months to 1–2 years—the muscle fibers undergo permanent degenerative changes, and eventually they are replaced by connective and fat tissue. If all the motor units of a muscle are affected simultaneously by denervation, the entire muscle degenerates at an even rate. In many disease processes, however, individual motor units may degenerate by denervation while others remain intact. In this case the surviving motor units become hypertrophic and develop sprouts into denervated neighboring units which in this fashion become recipients of a new nerve supply. As a result, muscles which have undergone partial denervation contain a smaller number of functioning motor units, but many of them may be very large because of sprouting, and their fibers may be hypertrophic. Clinically this sprouting can be detected by the appearance of giant motor-unit potentials in the electromyogram. Sprouting is type-specific. Type I fibers grow sprouts only into degenerating Type I fibers, and denervated Type II fibers can be reinnervated only from other surviving Type II fibers. As a result in a partially denervated muscle the fibers are grouped according to type, while in a healthy muscle Type I and Type II fibers are mixed randomly in checkerboard fashion.

A muscle which has been made inactive by splinting, by section of its tendon, or by upper motor neuron disease undergoes similar changes, but the loss of bulk rarely exceeds 30–35 percent of normal. Disuse atrophy causes a preferential atrophy of the fast-twitch Type II fibers. The same is true for upper-motor-neuron lesions that have caused spasticity or rigidity.[13–15]

The muscle atrophy of immobilization is entirely due to a decrease in fiber size. There is no decrease in the number of fibers. Cardenas et al. have shown that earlier reports to the contrary were based on faulty techniques.[16] These authors immobilized the hind legs of rats in plaster casts; after 4 weeks, the number of muscle fibers was identical with those of controls. The tensile strength and energy absorption capacity of an immobilized muscle decline rapidly.[17] This process is completely reversible once the immobilizing plaster cast has been removed. The relationship of the length of the muscle while immobilized to the extent of its atrophy has been a subject of investigation. Goldspink has shown recently that muscles react very differently when immobilized in a shortened or lengthened position.[18] The shortened immobilized muscle undergoes rapid atrophy and exhibits net losses of tissue protein because of a marked decrease in protein synthesis. Muscles immobilized in a lengthened position grow, compared to controls, and show increased rates of protein synthesis. This observation, if confirmed in humans, may have important clinical implications. If the same phenomenon holds true for immobilized human muscle, orthopedists may want to modify their methods of applying splints and casts by putting muscles on stretch, in order to avoid disuse atrophy.

Müller in his excellent review on the influence of training and inactivity on muscle strength reported that an immobilized muscle loses approximately 3 percent of its original strength per day.[19] He also noted that the strength of a muscle immobilized in a plaster cast declined in a linear fashion for the first 7 days. Thereafter, little strength was lost for the remaining period of immobilization. Müller suggests that the subjects learn to perform unintentional isometric contractions within the cast which prevent further loss of strength.

Contractures.   A muscle that is immobilized in a shortened position becomes contracted. This condition is reversible for a limited period of time. Eventually, much of the muscle substance is replaced by fibrous tissue, and normal length and function cannot be restored. Certain neuromuscular diseases predispose to the development of contractures. They are particularly common in poliomyelitis, Duchenne's muscular dystrophy, and other chronic spinal and muscular atrophies. More commonly yet, contractures develop as a result of an immobilization in a fixed position. A patient who, for whatever reason, is unable to walk or stand and who spends much of the time sitting in a chair may develop contractures of the hip flexor muscles. At a later date, when he tries to walk again, he will be unable to extend his hip. He has to walk over a flexed hip joint, and in order to keep the center of gravity over the supporting foot, he also needs to keep the knee in flexion. Obviously this makes for a fatiguing, awkward, and unsafe gait. Hip flexor contractures are easily overlooked since the motion of the pelvis can obscure the inability to extend the hip. The Thomas maneuver, by which the opposite hip is held in flexion over the abdomen, stabilizes the pelvis and brings a deficit of hip extension to light. Hip flexor contractures are also commonly seen in above-knee amputees who spend much of their time sitting in a wheelchair and who put a pillow under their stump while in bed.

Knee flexor contractures have a similar mechanism but are more easily detected. Heel cord contractures are common in bedridden patients who are allowed to lie with their ankles in plantar flexion. Ischemia of the limb accelerates the development of muscle contractures. The management of contractures is discussed in Chapter 5.

THE MANAGEMENT OF ATROPHIC AND DENERVATED MUSCLES

When a limb is immobilized during the treatment of an injury, the muscles become weak and atrophic. Once the need for immobilization has passed, muscle bulk and strength can be restored by therapeutic exercises. Exercise increases the volume of muscle fibers but not their numbers. It reverses the pathologic process of disuse atrophy.

Muscle fibers become hypertrophic only when stressed sufficiently. The resumption of normal activities may be adequate to restore muscle bulk and strength, but the progress will be slow. It can be accelerated by stressing the muscle beyond its level of ordinary activity. The exercises may be isotonic (dynamic) or isometric (static). A great variety of exercise programs has been designed to correct disuse atrophy. Their common denominator is a step-wise increase of the load until the desired goal has been reached. A system of progressive resistive exercises was developed by

De Lorme.[20] The muscle lifts a light load ten times, through the full range of motion of the joint. The load is then increased, and the muscle lifts this new load ten times through full range. Eventually, after successive increases, the maximal load which a muscle can lift ten times in succession will be reached. This is called "the 10 repetition maximum." This procedure is repeated daily. After one week, a new and higher repetition maximum load is determined. The program continues in this fashion until the desired muscle strength has been achieved. Various authors have developed modifications that simplify this rather complicated program. Müller reported that one near-maximal contraction per day held for 6 sec causes a significant increase of strength.[19] Five daily maximal contractions at 6 sec each produced the best results. A system of brief maximal exercise was described by Rose.[21] The quadriceps femoris in his experimental set-up lifts a maximal load once a day from 90 degrees of knee flexion to full extension and then holds the load in an isometric contraction for 5 sec. The load is increased every day by small increments. Once the maximal strength is reached, it can be maintained at this level by one brief maximal exercise session once a week.

Isometric exercises may be preferred if the joint is painful and inflamed and should not be stressed. The muscle holds the weight in a static contraction without effecting a joint motion. In our hands isokinetic exercises have been particularly effective in retraining weakened muscles, since they impose an even load on the muscle throughout the entire arc of motion.[6] However, isokinetic exercises require special equipment which is not universally available.

A partially denervated muscle is capable of contracting in response to volitional impulses but the force of contraction is diminished. Whether a partially denervated muscle can be strengthened by exercises or whether it will be actually harmed by fatiguing stresses is still not clear. Müller and Beckmann studied the effect of training on unused paretic muscles in children with birth injuries or poliomyelitis. About half of the muscles could be trained to at least one half of the strength of the corresponding normal muscle on the other side of the body.[22] They concluded that at least 80 percent of the fibers had been intact but by habit had remained inactive and therefore developed disuse weakness. Children with paralyses due to birth injuries did much better than those who had been afflicted by poliomyelitis.

Bennett and Knowlton, on the other hand, reported five cases of poliomyelitis and traumatic quadriplegia in which partially denervated muscles became weaker from overuse.[23] The authors coined the term of "overwork weakness," and they warned that the damage may be permanent. The normal individual is protected against overworking his muscles by the accumulation of metabolic end products which engender a sensation of fatigue and discomfort. The circulation cannot keep up with the metabolic demands of excessive effort, a limiting and protective factor against overwork. This mechanism is not operative in a muscle damaged by poliomyelitis. The ratio of blood supply to the remaining muscle fibers is greater than in the normal muscle and for this reason metabolic end products do not accumulate and do not set a natural limit. Much earlier Sherrington had postulated that the myoneural junction acted as a fuse protecting muscle fibers against overwork.[24] An overload, according to his hypothesis, stops the transmission of impulses at the myoneural junction, thereby protecting the motor unit from the noxious effects of overactivity. The validity of this concept is uncertain.

In practice, exercises should be prescribed cautiously, if

muscle weakness is due to injury or neurologic disease. The effect of exercise must be gauged carefully by repeated muscle testing. A muscle has been stressed excessively if it is weaker after a bout of exercise than before. This is particularly true when the increased weakness is still present on the following day. We have been impressed by the observation that patients with neuropathies are often stronger on Mondays, when they have had a respite of two days from "therapeutic" exercise, than on any other day of the week. There is no evidence that exercise improves the muscle function of patients with acute polyneuritis, and most neurologist will agree that these patients are best treated with rest. Once the acute phase has passed a cautiously administered program of excercise carefully supervised by the physician may be tried.

Electrotherapy. Totally denervated muscles no longer respond to stimuli arising in the central nervous system. They lose tone, become flaccid, and undergo degenerative changes which eventually become permanent. However, they contract upon electrical stimulation, and there is adequate evidence that contractions induced by electrical impulses retard or possibly even prevent degeneration. Electrotherapy, therefore, is indicated if there is any expectation that reinnervation may take place in some weeks or months. Therapeutic electrical stimulation finds its most common application in lower motor neuron lesions caused by injury of the nerve, toxins, or disease. In poliomyelitis, for instance, anterior horn cells may recover, or muscle fibers may receive a new nerve supply by sprouts from intact neighboring motor units. In this case, it may be well to maintain the functional capacity of the muscle fiber by frequent electrical stimulation. Electrotherapy is not useful in myopathic muscle weakness or in lesions of the myoneural junction.

Therapeutic electrical stimulation may also be indicated in lesions of the central nervous system. While the motor unit is intact, it receives no stimuli through natural pathways, and for this reason it may undergo disuse atrophy. Electrical stimuli will make the muscle contract and provide the means of active exercise, which cannot be achieved in any other way.

A motor unit responds to electrical stimulation only at moments when the current abruptly changes strength or direction. A steadily flowing direct current causes a contraction only at the moments of closing and opening, this is, when it begins and ceases to flow. A current in order to induce muscle contractions, therefore, must either be an alternating current, or it must consist of rapid unidirectional short impulses. The most commonly used therapeutic current consists of pulses that reach their peak almost instantaneously and have a duration of about 1 msec. The current strength varies from 1 to 30 mA.

Nerve fibers are more responsive to electrical stimuli than muscle fibers. Therefore, if the nerve is intact it will respond to an electrical impulse and effect a muscle contraction at a threshold much lower than would be required for the direct stimulation of muscle fibers. The threshold is a function of the duration of the pulse and the current intensity, measured in volts or milliamperes. An intact nerve fiber responds to electrical impulses of a duration of 1–100 msec at the same threshold of current intensity, which is called the rheobase. Impulses of shorter duration than, e.g., 1 msec, require a higher current intensity to cause the muscle to contract. At still shorter impulse durations, the needed current intensity becomes so great as to be painful. The relationship of current intensity to impulse duration needed to make a muscle contract is plotted as the "strength–duration curve" (Figure 5). It is used as a diagnostic test for denervation.

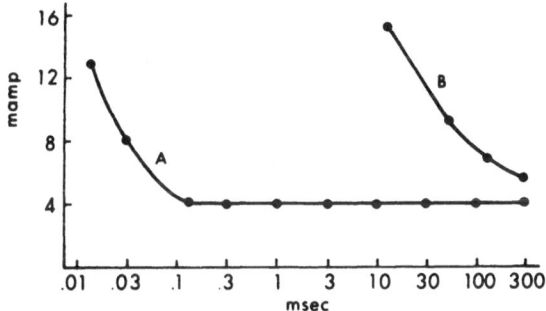

FIGURE 5. Strength–duration curve. A: Normal muscle. B: Denervated muscle.

When the nerve is damaged by disease or injury, it no longer reacts to electrical impulses. If both pulse duration and current intensity are increased sufficiently, the muscle fibers respond directly but at a much higher threshold. Muscle fibers require pulses of about 100-msec duration, about 100 times as much as when the impulse is mediated through an intact nerve. The threshold of current intensity is also higher. When a muscle is stimulated through its nerve, the contraction is brisk and forceful. When the muscle fiber is stimulated directly, it responds with a sluggish slow contraction of lesser force.

The frequency of the impulses is also of considerable importance. If the frequency is low, the muscle relaxes completely in between stimuli. As the impulses follow each other more rapidly, there is less and less time for relaxation between contractions. Eventually, at frequencies of 20/sec, when the nerve is intact, the contractions fuse so that there is no relaxation at all, and a tetanic contraction results. The muscle remains contracted until the current flow is stopped. A denervated muscle fuses single twitches to a tetanic contraction at frequencies as low as 5–10 per second. Yet, as mentioned before, the contraction remains sluggish.

In clinical practice a normally innervated muscle can be therapeutically stimulated by a variety of currents. The individual impulses should have a short rise time; square wave currents are used most often. The frequency should be high enough to produce a forceful tetanic contraction. The duration of each impulse may be short (approximately 1 msec), the current intensity is adjusted to need and patient comfort. The denervated muscle is ideally stimulated by currents with frequencies of 5–30 per second and current durations of at least 100 msec. The intensity is adjusted to need.

It has been shown that denervated muscles must be stimulated two to three times a day in order to prevent atrophy and degeneration. For this reason we teach our patients to administer electrical stimulation to themselves. The patient is supplied with a small battery-powered stimulator to take home. The apparatus generates a direct current which is closed and broken with a hand-operated switch. The muscle is stimulated each time the current is closed. The cathode is used as the active electrode.

THE MANAGEMENT OF IMMOBILIZATION RESULTING FROM MUSCLE PARALYSIS

The management of paralyzed patients begins with a thorough assessment of the extent and distribution of muscle weakness and its effects on the overall function of the individual. Whatever activity can be achieved by corrective measures will be of a great advantage to the patient psychologically and physically. It will prevent or at least retard the disastrous effects of immobilization. This principle holds true even when the long-term prognosis for survival is poor. Vignos has shown that continued ambulation with braces significantly improves the life expectancy of children with Duchenne's muscular dystrophy.[25] Paralyzed patients, regardless of the nature of their illness, deserve to be kept active and alive as long as possible. Even though the physician may not be able to cure the underlying disease, efforts must be expended to help the patient adjust to his disability, physically and emotionally.

Braces can be effective substitutes for absent muscle function. Modern bracing (or orthotics) is based on sound principles of biomechanics. The more distal and the more limited the paralysis the easier and more successful will be the brace application. A foot drop, whether caused by a peripheral nerve lesion or by a stroke, is easily managed by appropriate bracing. The conventional brace has two steel bars which are attached to a cuff located below the knee. The joint of the brace is aligned with the ankle joint. The distal part of the brace attaches to the heel of the shoe. The shoe must have a steel plate incorporated into the sole in order to provide leverage action. The brace joint may contain a spring. The plantar flexion action of the ankle stretches the spring. Once the tension is released, the spring snaps the ankle into a position of dorsiflexion. In this fashion the spring acts as a substitute for nonfunctioning muscles. Depending on circumstances, pins are used instead of the springs. They hold the foot in a fixed position, usually at a 90-degree angle to the leg. This arrangement reduces mobility but provides more stability. By leverage action it also keeps the knee joint from collapsing or snapping into hyperextension if knee extensors or flexors are weak. Lightweight plastic braces with posterior calf shells and a foot plate worn in a shoe are available and often preferred. When the knee needs to be braced directly, the upright bars extend to below the groin. The mechanical knee joint is furnished with a manual lock which the patient opens when he wants to sit; in the standing position the orthotic knee is locked and keeps the knee joint from collapsing (Figure 6). Bracing can be carried higher to support the hips and portions of the spine. Very extensive bracing, however, is often not accepted by the patient. Application and removal are time consuming and tiring, and walking with bulky and heavy braces carries with it a high energy cost. Many paraplegic patients who have been braced and have become proficient brace walkers while hospitalized in a rehabilitation department discard their braces after they return home and rely on wheelchair locomotion.[26]

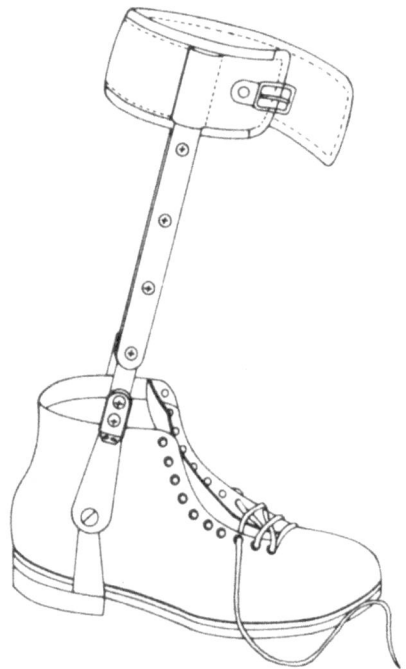

FIGURE 6. Below-knee brace with double-action orthotic ankle joint.

A variety of splints are used for paralyzed upper extremities. Static splints hold a given joint in a functional position and substitute for those muscles which usually act a stabilizers. For instance, when the wrist extensors are paralyzed, a lightweight plastic splint holds the wrist in a slightly extended position. This allows the fingers to function, or if their muscles are paralyzed also, it permits the use of adaptive devices clipped to the hand. Dynamic splints effect substitute movements. For instance, in patients quadriplegic at C6-7 level, the wrist extensors are intact, but all muscles supplying the fingers are paralyzed. A tenodesis splint holds the thumb opposed to the first two fingers. When the patient extends the wrist, the leverage action of the splint draws the second and third finger to the thumb in a functionally forceful pinch grasp (Figure 7).

The foregoing examples are only given to illustrate the principles of bracing. For details the reader is referred to monographs on orthotics.[27,28] In general, the prescription of a brace must be carefully considered in light of the patient's needs. The best results will be obtained if physician, therapists, and orthotists cooperate in designing and prescribing the appropriate device. Braces should not be prescribed unless they fulfill a real need and enhance the pa-

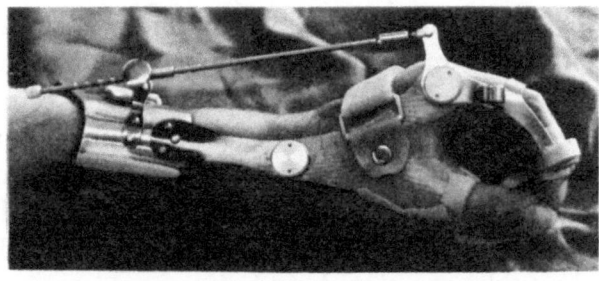

FIGURE 7. Tenodesis hand–wrist splint.

tient's overall function. The device should be as simple in design as possible so patient and family can apply it without undue difficulty. It should be as light in weight as possible and acceptable in appearance. The patient's concepts of cosmetic acceptability are often at variance with those of physician and brace maker. For this reason it is important to show the patient at least a picture of the brace before it is manufactured. Patients simply will not use a device which in their eyes is disfiguring.

Functional Electrical Stimulation. The use of electrical stimulators to produce functional movements has been made possible by the development of lightweight small transistor units. The first functional stimulator was developed by Liberson in 1961 for the management of patients with foot drop due to strokes.[29] The active electrode was applied over the peroneal nerve just below the knee. A switch was placed in the shoe. When the patient lifted the foot off the ground the circuit was closed and the electric stimulator effected a dorsiflexor motion of the ankle. When the foot was planted onto the ground the switch interrupted the current. This device never became popular. The current was uncomfortable and most patients rejected the stimulator after a short trial.

Functional electrical stimulation is possible only for muscles weakened or paralyzed by an upper motor neuron lesion. In this condition the motor unit from the anterior horn cell to the muscle fiber is intact but the muscle is paralyzed because it receives no stimuli from the central nervous system. Because the peripheral motor unit is intact the muscle can respond to short duration currents of tolerable intensity with a contraction that is forceful enough to be utilized for functional purposes. On the other hand, a denervated muscle, as pointed out before, requires currents of higher intensity and longer duration, and the resulting contraction is sluggish and lacks the force necessary for functional utilization. The indications for functional electrical stimulation, therefore, are cerebral or spinal-cord lesions.

The correction of foot drop has remained the main application for the use of functional stimulators. At Rancho Los Amigos in Downey, California, the electrodes are surgically implanted over the peroneal nerve. Less current is required since the nerve is stimulated directly, without the interposition of subcutaneous tissue. As in Liberson's early model the switch is placed in the shoe. The current consists of square wave pulses with a duration of 20 μsec and a frequency of 33 Hz (33 impulses per second). The voltage is adjustable to need and varies from 0.4 to 0.8 volts. Net current flow which would cause tissue damage by changes in ion concentration is prevented by inductive coupling of the stimulator, so that an equal amount of current will flow in the opposite direction in between pulses. A cyclic module can be attached to the transmitter, which provides an automatic 5-sec stimulation followed by 30 sec of rest. When the cyclic module is in operation the equipment can be used to stimulate the nerve and exercise the muscle at times when the patient is not walking. The stimulator selectively activates the tibialis anterior muscle. This unfortunately leads to an imbalanced ankle dorsiflexion, that is, the ankle inverts while it flexes. In order to provide for a more balanced motion it is necessary to also give some stimulation to the evertors of the ankle. The Rancho Los Amigos group is now working on this problem. A similar system can be used to functionally stimulate a weak or paralyzed quadriceps group.[30]

Electrical stimulators have been designed to provide grasp and release to hands paralyzed by quadriplegia. Peckham and Mortimer have summarized the requirements for such a device: The grasp must have adequate strength. The muscles must be resistant to fatigue, since contractions have to be maintained for many minutes. The contraction must be smooth, which means that fused (tetanic) contractions have to be achieved. The degree of contractile force must be variable and subject to the patient's volitional control.[31,32] These requirements are difficult to meet. Peckham and Mortimer insert electrodes into the finger flexors and extensors. The wrist is stabilized by a lightweight splint. The stimulator allows for the delivery of impulses in sequence and permits the adjustment of pulse width and frequency. The patient controls the stimulator by alternately depressing and elevating the shoulder girdle.

The functional electrical stimulation of the quadriplegic hand has not yet advanced past the state of investigation. Considerable problems stand in the way of general clinical application. Some of these difficulties need to be discussed. First of all, electrically induced muscle contractions differ considerably from physiologic contractions. Under normal circumstances different motor units are activated in alternation and contract asynchronously, which makes for smooth overall muscle contractions and protects the individual motor units from fatigue. Electrical stimuli activate the same motor units over and over again. They fire in synchrony and fatigue rapidly. Second, at frequencies needed to produce fused contractions the intramuscular vessels are occluded by the contracting muscle fibers, and this obviously interferes with the supply of needed oxygen. Peckham and Mortimer are trying to overcome this particular problem by the use of sequential stimulators which activate different portions of the muscle at different times. Finally, the order in which different motor units are activated by electricity is the reverse of the physiologic activation process. Under normal conditions small diameter fibers of the slow-twitch fatigue-resistant motor units are activated first and before the large-diameter fast-twitch glycolytic fibers which are fatigue prone are activated. Large diameter fibers, however, have the lowest threshold to electrical stimulation, and, for this reason, they will respond first, while the fatigue-resistant fibers have the highest threshold and, furthermore, are in the interior of the muscle and farther removed from the stimulating electrode. As a result, fatigue sets in early and makes it impossible to sustain contractions long enough to perform functional tasks. There is evidence in animal experiments that fatigue-prone glycolytic fast-twitch fibers can be converted to fatigue-resistant oxidative fibers by prolonged electrical stimulation.[4,33,34] It remains to be seen whether these observations will be applicable to the human.

The use of functional electric stimulators requires good cognitive functions and a high level of motivation. If proprioception is affected by the disease a feedback mechanism must be provided which the patient must learn to use. It is obvious that patients must be carefully selected, and even then rejections will be common. The gadget tolerance of individuals is limited. The achievements of electronic engineering often surpass the psychologic capabilities of human beings.

LOCOMOTION OF THE SEVERELY PARALYZED PATIENT

A patient who is unable to walk can retain a fair degree of independence by the use of a wheelchair. The modern wheelchair is collapsible so that it can be folded and carried in an automobile. It has 24-inch wheels in the rear and 8-inch casters in front. The large wheels are equipped with hand-rims which the patient uses to propel the chair. If the pa-

tient's hands are weak, knobs are added to the rims to facilitate the propulsion. Brakes on the rear wheels are standard
equipment. Wheelchairs have stationary or removable foot
rests. Elevating footrests are used if one or both legs need to
be elevated. Armrests are either stationary or removable. In a
patient with paralysis of both lower extremities, removable
sidearms must be used so the patient can slide in and out of
the chair sideways. Patients need to use both arms to propel
the chair in order to keep it moving in a straight line. However, many hemiplegic patients with one paralyzed upper
extremity learn to propel and steer their chair with their
sound arm and sound leg. Chairs with one-arm drives which
can be propelled and steered with one arm are available.

A wheelchair prescription must consider the various
facets of the patient's disability and special equipment
should be ordered accordingly. Physicians and physical
therapists should prescribe the components so the chair will
be as useful as possible to the patient. Families should be
discouraged from buying a wheelchair at the corner
drugstore without first consulting physician or therapist.

Once the chair has been obtained the physical therapist
will train the patient in its use. The therapist will also teach
the patient how to transfer in and out of the chair to a bed, a
toilet, or an automobile. The transfer technique to be used
depends on the strength of the upper extremities. If the
upper extremities are paralyzed, family members are taught
how to lift the patient without undue stresses on their own
backs. Hydraulic lifts are available if it is not possible to lift
the patient manually. In the absence of medical indications,
no patient should be confined to bed just because he or she is
paralyzed.

A patient who cannot propel a wheelchair can be furnished with a motorized chair. These chairs are powered by

rechargeable batteries. The motor is activated by the patient with a switch or jog stick which is also used to steer the chair. The manual force required to operate the controls is minimal. Other controls are available if the upper extremities are completely paralyzed. Chairs can be operated by depressing the switch with the chin. If the neck motion is also limited the patient can still operate the controls by breathing in and out of a tube which connects to a switching mechanism, the so-called "sip and puff" controls. More recently eye-controlled wheelchairs have been developed. The patient wears a special pair of glasses and can propel, stop, and steer the chair by turning the eyes in one direction or the other.

Complex systems of this type will be useful to patients who are motivated to retain independence in spite of their overwhelming handicap and who are skillful enough to learn the use of the intricate controls. Too often, elaborate equipment is prescribed and then rejected by the patient because it surpasses his gadget tolerance. The recent advances in engineering are impressive, but the human factor remains paramount.

REFERENCES

1. Walton, J. N. *Disorders of Voluntary Muscle.* 3rd Ed., Chapter 1. Edinburgh and London, 1974. Churchill Livingstone.
2. Armstrong, R. B. Energy release in the extrafusal muscle fiber. *Neuromuscular Mechanism for Therapeutic and Conditioning Exercise* (H. G. Knuttgen, ed.). Baltimore, 1976. University Park Press.
3. Ianuzzo, C. D. The cellular composition of human skeletal muscle. In: *Neuromuscular Mechanism for Therapeutic and Conditioning Excercise* H. G. Knuttgen, ed.). Baltimore 1976. University Park Press.
4. Riley, D. A., and Allin, E. F. The effects of inactivity, programmed stimulation, and denervation on the histochemistry of skeletal muscle fiber types. *Exp. Neurol.* **40**:391, 1973.

5. Brunnstrom, S. *Clinical Kinesiology*, Chapter 2. Philadelphia, 1962. F. A. Davis Co.
6. Thistle, H. G., Hislop, H. J., Moffroid, M., and Lowman, E. W. Isokinetic contraction: New concept of resistive exercise. *Arch. Phys. Med. Rehab.* **48**:279, 1967.
7. Duchenne, G. B. *Physiology of Motion (1867)*. Translated by E. B. Kaplan. Philadelphia, 1949. J. B. Lippincott Co.
8. Close, J. R. *Motor Function in the Lower Extremities*. 2nd Ed. Springfield, Illinois, 1973. Charles C Thomas.
9. Basmajan, J. V. *Muscles Alive*. 4th Ed. Baltimore, 1978. Williams & Wilkins.
10. Kendall, H. O., Kendall, F. P., and Wadsworth, G. E. *Muscle Testing and Function*. 2nd Ed. Baltimore, 1971. Williams & Wilkins.
11. Daniels, L., and Worthingham, C. *Muscle Testing*. 3rd Ed. Philadelphia, 1972. W. B. Saunders.
12. Nathan, P. W. Intrathecal phenol to relieve spasticity in paraplegia. *Lancet* **2**:1099, 1959.
13. Mayer, R. F., Burke, R. E., and Kanda, K. Immobilization and muscle atrophy. *Trans. Am. Neurol. Assoc.* **101**:145, 1976.
14. Engel, K. A critique of congenital myopathies and other disorders. In: *Exploratory Concepts of Muscular Disorders*. Amsterdam, 1966. Excerpta Medica Foundation.
15. Edström, L., and Kugelberg, E. Histochemical composition, distribution of fibers and fatigability of single motor units. *J. Neurol. Neurosurg. Psychiatry* **31**:424, 1968.
16. Cardenas, D. D., Stolov, W. C., and Hardy, R. Muscle fiber numbers in immobilization atrophy. *Arch. Phys. Med. Rehab.* **58**:423, 1977.
17. Järvinen, M. Immobilization effect on the tensile properties of striated muscle: An experimental study in the rat. *Arch. Phys. Med. Rehab.* **58**:123, 1977.
18. Goldspink, D. F. The influence of immobilization and stretch on protein turnover of rat skeletal muscle. *J. Physiol.* **264**:267, 1977.
19. Müller, E. A. Influence of training and of inactivity on muscle strength. *Arch. Phys. Med. Rehab.* **51**:449, 1970.
20. DeLorme, T. L., and Watkins, A. L. Technics of progressive resistance exercise. *Arch. Phys. Med. Rehab.* **29**:263, 1948.
21. Rose, D. L., Radzyminski, S. F., and Beatty, R. R. Effect of brief maximal exercise on the strength of the quadriceps femoris. *Arch. Phys. Med. Rehab.* **38**:157, 1957.
22. Müller, E. A., and Beckmann, H. Die Trainierbarkeit von Kindern mit gelähmten Muskeln durch isometrische Kontraktionen. *Z. Orthop.* **102**:139, 1966.

23. Bennett, R. L., and Knowlton, G. C. Overwork weakness in partially denervated skeletal muscles. *Clin. Orthop.* **12**:22, 1958.
24. Sherrington, C. S. Observation on the scratch reflex in the spinal dog. *J. Physiol.* **34**:1, 1906.
25. Vignos, P. J., Spencer, G. E., and Archibald, K. C. Management of progressive muscular dystrophy of childhood. *J. Am. Med. Assoc.* **184**:89, 1963.
26. Hussey, R. W. and Stauffer, E. S. Spinal cord injury. Requirements for ambulation. *Arch. Phys. Med. Rehab.* **54**:544, 1973.
27. Licht, S. *Orthotics*. New Haven, 1966. Elizabeth Licht.
28. *Atlas of Orthotics*. American Academy of Orthopedic Surgeons. St. Louis, 1975. C. V. Mosby.
29. Liberson, W. T., Holmquest, H. J., Scot, D., and Dow, M. Functional electrotherapy: Stimulation of the peroneal nerve synchronized with the swing phase of the gait of hemiplegic patients. *Arch. Phys. Med. Rehab.* **42**:101, 1961.
30. Waters, R. Electrical stimulation of the peroneal and femoral nerves in man. In: *Functional Electrical Stimulation. Applications in Neural Prostheses. Biomedical Engineering and Instrumentation,* Vol. 3 (F. T. Hambrecht and J. B. Reswick, eds.). New York and Basel, 1977. Marcel Dekker.
31. Mortimer, J. T., and Peckham, P. H. Intramuscular electrical stimulation. In: *Neural Organization and Its Relevance to Prosthetics* (W. S. Fields and L. A. Leavitt, eds). New York, 1973. Intercontinental Medical Book Corp.
32. Peckham, P. H., and Mortimer, J. T. Restoration of hand function in the quadriplegic through electrical stimulation. In: *Functional Electrical Stimulation. Applications in Neural Prostheses. Biomedical Engineering and Instrumentation,* Vol. 3 (F. T. Hambrecht and J. B. Reswick, eds.). New York and Basel, 1977. Marcel Dekker.
33. Peckham, P. H., Mortimer, J. T., and Van Der Meulen, J. P. Physiologic and metabolic changes in white muscle of cat following induced exercise. *Brain Res.* **50**:424, 1973.
34. Pette, D., Ramirez, B. U., Müller, W., Simon, R., Exner, G. U., and Hildebrand, R. Influence of intermittent long-term stimulation on contractile, histochemical and metabolic properties of fibre populations in fast and slow rabbit muscles. *Pfluegers Arch. Eur. J. Physiol.* **361**:1, 1975.

CHAPTER 5

The Immobilization of Joints

The joint is an organ of motion; its structural and functional integrity is predicated on motility. The deleterious effects of immobility are based on the structure and biomechanics of joints. The deep layers of the cartilage are nourished by the blood vessels of the subchondral bone, but the superficial layers are dependent on the synovial fluid for their nutrition. The synovial fluid is viscous and has a high surface tension, which makes it cling to the cartilage. Joint motion makes for a constant interchange of fluid between the surface layers of the articular cartilage and the synovial fluid. When the joint is immobile the flow of the synovial fluid ceases, and the diffusion of fluid in and out of the cartilage stops. Joint motion causes alternating cartilage compression and distention. Absence of these pressure fluctuations causes a stagnation of the intercellular fluid of the cartilage and decreases its nutrition. After some period of time degenerative changes become permanent.

The effect of immobilization on joints has been studied experimentally.[1,2] After prolonged immobilization, contractures of the joint capsule and especially of periarticular muscles are responsible for much of the restriction of motion. Within the joint cavity connective tissue proliferates and causes adhesions which significantly contribute to a further limitation of motion. The abnormal joint function damages the cartilage. The matrix shows fibrillar degeneration. Ulcerations and clefts form in those areas where the joint surfaces are in contact and especially when they are firmly compressed by muscle contractures. The degeneration of the cartilage is not reversible.

Mathias and Glupe immobilized the knees of rabbits in a position of extreme flexion.[2] After 4 weeks, the joints appeared drier than normal. The cartilage was thinner and began to show ulcerations in those areas where cartilagenous surfaces were in contact and under pressure. After 8–12 weeks, the degeneration of cartilage in the pressure zones had further advanced, and some thinning had also appeared in those areas which were not under pressure. Under the pressure zones the subchondral bone showed signs of atrophy. Connective tissue was proliferating into the joint cavity. After 12 weeks, the periarticular ligaments had become slack, and this had diminished the lateral stability of the joint. The menisci showed fibrillar degeneration and the formation of fissures. The authors also measured the space between the articulating bones in radiographs of human subjects in whom a normal hip had to be immobilized in a spica cast. The spaces showed a progressive diminution. This was more marked in young individuals, probably because the cartilage is better hydrated to begin with and, therefore, subject to a greater water loss and more extensive shrinkage.

Enneking and Horowitz reported ten cases in which human knee joints had been immobilized for 13 to 20 months.[3] Their pathologic data were similar to those obtained in animal experiments. The periarticular tissues were contracted. The joint cavity was eventually obliterated by fibrofatty connective tissue. This tissue apparently originates from the infrapatellar fat pad, the suprapatellar pouch, and the posterior recesses of the joint. It fills the joint cavity, envelops the cruciate ligaments, and attaches to unopposed cartilagenous surfaces. Eventually the cartilage is replaced by the fibrofatty tissue which penetrates to the subchondral bone. In areas where the articular surfaces were in contact the cartilage became fibrillated and showed a cystic degeneration. The articular surfaces became fused to each other by fibrous connective tissue and in some places by endochondral ossification. There was, however, no gross evidence of bony ankylosis. The authors concluded that the intraarticular changes play a major role in the restriction of motion of immobilized joints. After they had divided the extraarticular ligaments and muscles a significant limitation of motion remained, obviously due to the formation of connective tissue in the joint cavity. It should be pointed out that in Enneking's study the immobilization had been present for a very long period of time. However, similar changes have been observed after much shorter periods of immobilization. Thomas found that the extension stiffness of a healthy immobilized knee was initiated early by the agglutination of fluid in the upper recesses of the knee joint resulting from diminished synovial fluid exchange.[4] This eventually causes the formation of fibrous cords between the synovial surfaces, leading to a restriction of motion. If the knee is immobilized in 60 degrees of flexion, the upper recesses remain unfolded, and fluid agglutination and the development of fibrous cords are avoided.

Field and Hueston's findings are at variance with those of Evans and Mathias.[5] They examined the interphalangeal joints of two patients whose fingers had become immobilized by Dupuytren's contractures. The cartilage had become pitted and eroded in those areas where the joint surfaces did not touch. The cartilage was thin and vascular

connective tissue had proliferated into the cartilagenous surface. In areas where the joint surfaces were opposed the
cartilage had remained intact. Hall had reported similar findings in animal experiments.[6]

Immobilization is particularly destructive if the joint surfaces are under pressure.[2,7] Walcher and Stürz, in a detailed
experimental study, showed that immobilized joints under
pressure develop ossification of the cartilage if the immobilization lasts for a long period of time.[8] The greater the
pressure the more extensive is the ossification.

These observations have important clinical applications.
When it becomes necessary to immobilize a joint, pressure
on the joint surfaces should be avoided. Weight bearing on
knee joints immobilized in extension may therefore be contraindicated. Undue pressure may also be exerted by muscle
and connective tissue contractures or by muscle spasticity.
Joints, therefore, should be immobilized in positions in
which these factors are minimized. Incomplete immobilization is more noxious than complete fixation because it allows
abnormal lateral motions, which by friction damage the joint
surfaces.[2] A complete immobilization is probably achieved
only by internal fixation.

CLINICAL APPLICATIONS

The function of joints is evaluated by inspection, palpa-
tion, and the measurement of range of motion. These measurements are made with a goniometer, the arms of which
must have the appropriate length in order to assure maximal
accuracy. Even then a fairly large margin of error remains.
This subject has been extensively reviewed by Moore.[9] The
highest degree of accuracy is achieved by the method of

P. O. Williams which measures the distance of two points on each side of a joint and calculates the angle by the law of cosines.[10] The neutral resting positions of joints are designated as the zero baseline. Zero points, for instance, are the positions of extension of elbows, hips, and knees. Methods of joint range of motion measurements and normal values are given in a number of publications.[11,12]

Muscle paralysis is a frequent cause of joint immobilization. Contractures develop more rapidly if the muscles are spastic. Not only do spastic muscles undergo permanent shortening but they also add to the damage of the articular structures by exerting continuous pressure on opposing joint surfaces. The development of periarticular contractures is further enhanced by trauma, edema, and insufficient arterial circulation. The hips, knees, and ankles of patients with inadequate arterial blood flow become contracted rapidly because of the formation of dense connective tissue once the patient stops walking and unless range of motion exercises are given regularly.

At times joints must be immobilized in order to treat a trauma or an infection. If the joint is immobilized in an optimal position, if the joint surfaces are not under pressure, and if the immobilization does not extend past 4 weeks, no permanent damage may result. Recent evidence indicates that the complete immobilization of joints afflicted by rheumatoid arthritis actually prevents joint damage and promotes recovery.[13] Partridge et al., in an elegant study, demonstrated many years ago that knee joints in the acute phase of rheumatoid arthritis did best when completely immobilized in a plaster cast.[14]

An injury or a bacterial infection may make it necessary to immobilize a joint for a prolonged period of time. In such a case the joint may permanently lose mobility. If this risk has

to be assumed, the joint must be immobilized in such a position that its stiffness will least interfere with the overall function of the extremity. For instance, an elbow ankylosed in
full extension makes the arm useless for activities such as
eating, shaving, brushing of teeth, etc. The functional positions for immobilized joints are shown below.

Spine	Normal curves.
Shoulder	30 degrees of flexion, 45 degrees of abduction, 15 degrees of external rotation.
Elbow	100 degrees of flexion, midway between supination and pronation.
Wrist	35–45 degrees of extension. No lateral deviation.
Fingers	25 degrees of flexion at m.p. joints. Slight flexion of i.p. joints.
Hip	20 degrees of flexion, slight abduction, no rotation.
Knee	Almost complete extension.
Ankle	Neutral position.
Toes	Slight flexion at m.p. joints. Extension of i.p. joints.

PREVENTION AND MANAGEMENT OF JOINT LOSS OF MOTION

Preventive measures must consider the cause of immobilization. Obviously, a normal joint incidentally immobilized for the treatment of a fracture is less vulnerable
than a joint that has been injured or one that has been
afflicted by a bacterial infection. Rheumatoid arthritis is more
destructive to joints than degenerative arthritis, and mobility
is lost more easily. Infected or seriously injured joints may
have to be immobilized for extended periods at a risk of a

permanent loss of mobility. The opinions are still divided with regard to the management of the acutely inflamed rheumatoid joint. Most physicians prefer to immobilize the joint by splinting for most of the day but prescribe active assistive range of motion exercises twice a day in order to prevent stiffening. On the other hand, as pointed out before, a rheumatoid joint may be safely immobilized for up to 30 days without loss of function.[13,14] In keeping with Mathias' observations, immobilized joints are less likely to lose mobility permanently if weight bearing and pressures induced by muscular contractions are avoided.[2] Incomplete immobilization that allows abnormal lateral shearing motions can also be quite destructive.

If joints are inflamed, exercises are best preceded by heat application. Superficial heating by warm moist packs is safer than deep heat such as diathermy or ultrasound. Heat relieves pain and muscle spasms. Pain is alleviated because heat appears to reduce the pain perception and conduction in the nerve endings and peripheral nerves. Heat reduces spasms by decreasing the sensitivity of the muscle spindles to stretch.[15] Heat also increases the capillary blood flow and facilitates the absorption of exudates and edema fluid. Application of heat is contraindicated in the presence of ischemia and, probably, over malignant tumors.

Exercises to retain the range of motion of painful and inflamed joints must be gentle. To whatever extent possible, the patient should move the joint actively. The therapist supports the affected limb and assists the motion. The exercise will induce some pain. However, if the pain is very severe and persists for many hours thereafter, the joint has been unduly stressed. In the presence of an acute or chronic arthritis, the muscles rapidly become weak and atrophic. Because muscles have a stabilizing and shock absorbing effect

on the articular structures, it is important to restore strength
as best as possible. The therapist instructs the patient to
tense his muscles in isometric contractions. If the joint inflammation is no longer acute, isometric exercise programs
should be instituted. For instance, a patient with an arthritic
knee uses the quadriceps to hold a weight against gravity
after the therapist has manually extended the knee with the
weight attached above the ankle. In this fashion the stress on
the knee joint is minimized, while the muscle performs an
optimal strengthening exercise.

Attempts to restore range of motion may be undertaken
after the acute inflammation has subsided. If joint tightness
is caused by muscle contractures, it can be undertaken earlier. It may also be more vigorous, since muscles tolerate
stretching forces better than articular structures. Stretching
should be done by a trained therapist who will know how to
gauge the force of a stretch and who understands the underlying pathologic condition. Subluxated rheumatoid joints
cannot be restored to full range of motion, and overly vigorous attempts will further damage the periarticular ligaments.
Particular caution is indicated if the extremity is anesthetic.
Forceful stretching may do considerable damage to the soft
tissues, and an osteoporotic bone may be fractured. In paraplegic patients excessive stretching of tight hip joints may cause
bleeding into the periarticular tissues. This in turn may result
in soft tissue calcification and heterotopic bone formation.

Not all stiff joints need to be or should be stretched to
full range. A hemiplegic patient with a tight shoulder will
have no functional benefit from fully restoring the range of
motion if the extremity has remained paralyzed. Many hours
can be wasted in a painful procedure which will be of no
benefit in the long run. To the quadriplegic patient a slight
stiffening of the small finger joints in flexion is a functional

advantage. If the hip extensors are paralyzed, a tightness of these muscles offers a functional benefit, and they should not be stretched. Bennett's statement that "no bodily segment should be mobilized unless the underlying strength of the musculature supporting this bodily segment is known" should always be kept in mind.[16]

On the other hand, restricted range of motion may seriously interfere with function. Hips and knees with extension deficit, for example, make for a cumbersome gait and increase the energy cost of walking.[17] In general, whether stretching of a contracted joint is indicated or contraindicated must be decided by those who understand body mechanics and are capable of anticipating the effect of increasing the mobility of a joint.

Stretching can be done manually. Prolonged stretching while applying a moderate force may be more effective than brief vigorous stretching. The elastic resistance of fibrous tissue is more easily overcome if the stretch is applied for a longer period of time. Spastic muscles particularly must be stretched slowly with a gradually increasing force, because a quick forceful jerking motion will elicit a stretch reflex, which is counterproductive. Heat application before stretching is beneficial, since heat alters the viscoelastic properties of tissues and makes them more pliable. At times a joint needs to be manipulated under anesthesia in order to improve mobility.

Special techniques are applied to some joints. Tight hip flexors are best stretched by weights over a pulley. The patient lies prone on a table, with the leg hanging over the edge supported by a sling at the distal end of the femur. The rope of the pulley is attached to the sling. For 20 min, 30–50 lb of weight are made to act on the tight hip. The pelvis is immobilized by a strap attached to the table (Figure 8). Tight

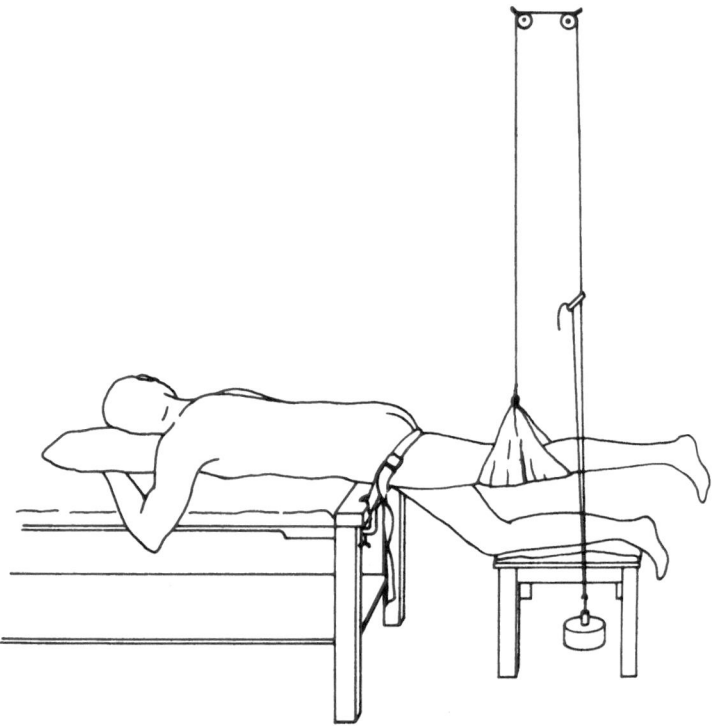

FIGURE 8. Stretching of hip flexion contracture by pulleys. Adapted with permission from F. H. Krusen, F. J. Kottke, and P. M. Ellwood, Jr., *Handbook of Physical Medicine and Rehabilitation*, 2nd Ed., W. B. Saunders, Philadelphia, 1971.

knee flexors are best stretched by 5- to 15-lb sandbags placed across the lower leg while the patient is prone. Another method consists of stretching the knee under anesthesia to the maximum extent and then applying a plaster cast in this position. The cast needs to be changed every 10–14 days. A few degrees of extension are gained with each cast change. It is usually not necessary to anesthetize the patient for the repeat cast applications. A pulley system applied through an exercise boot with weights attached is effective in stretching a tight heel cord. An exercise which can be done at home consists of having the patient stand at arm length from a wall with the foot on a wedge which raises the front of the foot. The patient then leans forward toward the wall for several minutes as tolerated.

A tight cervical spine is best stretched by traction. Traction applied to the lumbar spine is less effective, since it is more difficult to position the patient properly and to apply a force of sufficient magnitude.

The objective of stretching is to lengthen the fibrous connective tissue of the periarticular structures. The effect on the fibrofatty tissue within the joint cavity is more problematic. Enneking has observed that this tissue is firmly attached to the cartilage and that vigorous manipulations can cause an avulsion of pieces of cartilage.[3]

In summary, the stretching of tight joints is not to be undertaken lightly. Its indications and contraindications must be weighed carefully. The stretching should be done only by those who appreciate the possible complications and who know how much force to apply. At times stretching may have to be continued at home or in a nursing home by family members or nursing personnel. In that case the therapist should give careful instructions with return demonstration to ascertain that the procedure will be not only effective but also will do no harm.

REFERENCES

1. Evans, E. B., Eggers, G. W. N., Butler, J. K., and Blumel, J. Experimental immobilization and remobilization of rat knee joints. *J. Bone Jt. Surg.* **42A**:737, 1960.
2. Mathias, H. H. and Glupe, J. Immobilisation und Druckbelastung in

ihrer Wirkung auf die Gelenke. *Arch. Orthop. Unfall-Chir.* **60**:380, 1966.

3. Enneking, W. F., and Horowitz, M. The intra-articular effects of immobilization on the human knee. *J. Bone Jt. Surg.* **54A**:973, 1972.

4. Thomas, G. Die Strecksteife des Kniegelenkes. *Arch. Orthop. Unfall-Chir.* **60**:248, 1966.

5. Field, P. L. and Hueston, J. T. Articular cartilage loss in long-standing immobilisation of interphalangeal joints. *Br. J. Plastic Surg.* **23**:186, 1970.

6. Hall, M. C. Articular changes in the knee of the adult rat after prolonged immobilization in extension. *Clin. Orthop.* **34**:184, 1964.

7. Finsterbush, A., and Friedman, B. Reversibility of joint changes produced by immobilization in rabbits. *Clin. Orthop.* **111**:290, 1975.

8. Walcher, K. and Stürz, H. Führt Immobilisation und dosierte Druckbelastung eines Gelenkes im Tierversuch zum knöchernen Durchbau. *Arch. Orthop. Unfall-Chir.* **71**:216, 1971

9. Moore, M. L. Clinical assessment of joint motion. In: *Therapeutic Exercise*, 3rd Ed. (J. V. Basmajan, ed.), Chapter 6. Baltimore, 1978. Williams & Wilkins.

10. Williams, P. O. Assessment of mobility in joints. *Lancet* **2**:169, 1952.

11. American Medical Association, Committee on Rating of Mental and Physical Impairment. *Guides to the Evaluation of Permanent Impairment.* Chicago, 1971. American Medical Association.

12. American Academy of Orthopedic Surgeons. *Joint Motion, Method of Measuring and Recording.* Chicago, 1965. The Academy.

13. Smith, R. D., and Polley, H. F. Rest therapy for rheumatoid arthritis. *Mayo Clin. Proc.* **53**:141, 1978.

14. Partridge, R. E. H., and Duthie, J. J. R. Controlled trial on the effects of complete immobilization of the joint in rheumatoid arthritis. *Ann. Rheum. Dis.* **22**:91, 1963.

15. Lehmann, J. F., and DeLateur, B. J. Heat and cold in the treatment of arthritis. In: *Arthritis and Physical Medicine* (S. Licht, ed.). New Haven, 1969. Elizabeth Licht.

16. Bennett, R. L. Use and abuse of certain tools of physical medicine. *Arch. Phys. Med. Rehab.* **41**:485, 1960.

17. Kottke, F. J., and Kubicek, W. G. Relationship of the tilt of the pelvis to stable posture. *Arch. Phys. Med. Rehab.* **37**:81, 1956.

CHAPTER 6

The Effects of Immobilization on the Skin

One of the major hazards to face immobilized patients is the breakdown of the skin and underlying tissues. Those areas that are exposed to prolonged and excessive pressures are vulnerable, especially wherever bony prominences are close to the surface. Under normal conditions the skin is protected by frequent movements which shift the body weight from one area to the other. The immobilized patient is incapable of performing these weight shifts, and the same skin area remains under pressure for long periods of time.

Tissue breakdown occurs if the external pressure exceeds the capillary pressure for an extended span of time. The intracapillary pressure is approximately 25 mm Hg. Kosiak *et al.* measured pressures of 300 mm Hg and more under the ischial tuberosity in the sitting position.[1] Padding the seat with 2-inch foam rubber decreased the pressure to about one-half. Bush reported that the pressure under the tibial tuberosities was significantly greater when the feet were supported on the footrests of the wheelchair than when the legs were allowed to hang free.[2] In that position the pressure was distributed over a wider surface area, i.e., the posterior thighs. Lindan was able to measure the pressure over the skin surface of a recumbent man at more than 1000 points.[3] From his data he constructed isobars which outlined the pressure distribution over the entire body surface. In the supine position, the greatest pressures are over the sacrum, ischial tuberosities, heels, scapulae, elbows, and occiput. In the prone position maximal pressures are exerted on the patellae and anterior chest wall. In the lateral position the trochanter is particularly vulnerable. A harder surface increases the maximal pressure, the area of higher pressure contact, and the steepness of the isobar gradients. It decreases the area of lower-pressure contact. In addition to the degree of pressure, the time during which the skin is exposed to pressure is also of critical importance. Kosiak, experimenting with dogs, plotted pressure versus time of exposure.[4] The relationship followed a parabolic curve. A pressure of 500 mm Hg applied for 2 hr caused an ulceration, and a pressure of 150 mm Hg caused a skin breakdown when applied for 12 hr. All tissues under pressure points, epidermis, subcutaneous tissue, muscle, fascia, and bone were affected. There was a latent period of an average of 4½ days from the time that pressure had been applied until ulcerations appeared. In one case the latent period was as long as 9 days.

Factors other than compressive pressure may play an important part in the development of decubitus ulcers. Reichel postulated that significant shearing forces act on the tissues overlying the sacrum.[5] These forces are particularly destructive in paraplegic patients who are in bed in a halfway sitting position. In this position the body slides forward and downward against the sacral skin which remains in the same spot because of the friction between bed and skin. The shearing mechanism disrupts the deeper tissues and exerts its main effect on the superficial fascia. These forces place blood vessels under stretch and may cause multiple small vessel thromboses. The result is a dissection of tissues under the skin and necrosis. Dinsdale, working with paraplegic swine, found that their skin tolerated rather large pressures.[6] Friction, however, added significantly to the trauma, apparently by eroding the surface layers of the skin. With isotope circulation studies he demonstrated that the friction did not invoke an ischemic mechanism.

Many experimental studies demonstrate that interference with the capillary blood flow resulting from pressure is the most salient factor in the development of ulcers. At low perfusion pressures the capillary flow is unstable; it may cease or reverse directions. The first response to excessive pressure is a reactive hyperemia. This is a compensatory response to a temporary ischemia, and it protects the tissue against permanent damage. Because of this hyperemic response, tissues can tolerate rather large pressures, as long as they are applied for very brief periods of time. This explains why breakdowns do not occur in the normal person who shifts weight often enough to keep the period of pressure application to a minimum. Other factors contribute to the development of pressure sores. The accumulation of edema in the compressed tissue constitutes an additional hazard, because it inhibits the movement of nutrients and oxygen from the capillaries to the cells. Anemia is another contributing factor. Moolten reported that hypoalbuminemia was correlated with pressure sore formation, even though it is not clear whether the low serum albumin in his cases may not have been due to protein loss from the oozing sores.[7] In any case, malnutrition is an important risk factor. The soiling of skin with urine and feces and excessive perspiration contribute significantly to the formation of decubitus ulcers. Exton-Smith has devised a scoring system so physicians and nurses may quickly discover those patients who are at risk of developing pressure sores.[8] Factors such as physical and mental state, mobility, activity, and incontinence are assigned point values which add up to a total score. Anesthetic skin is particularly vulnerable. Investigators have postulated that sensory nerve fibers have a neurotrophic function and that ulcers form more readily in the anesthetic skin because of the loss of this function. However, the existence of such a neurotrophic element within the sensory nervous system has never been demonstrated. Therefore, it is safe to assume that the anesthetic skin is vulnerable because the patient does not feel the friction and irritation from, e.g., a wrinkled bedsheet, and does not shift position to protect the skin.

The early recognition of harmful pressure effects is vital. A reddening of the skin indicates reactive hyperemia. If it disappears within 30–60 min, one may assume that no tissue damage has ensued. If the area under pressure is white, then the ischemia has been more profound, and degenerative changes may already be present and possibly irreversible. An induration of the skin or blister formation indicates injury to the superficial and deeper layers of the epidermis. Very often the subcutaneous tissue and muscle are more extensively damaged than the outer layers of the epidermis. They may undergo necrosis while the skin shows only an insignificant degree of reddening and induration. The inexperienced observer may not realize the extent of the destruction that has already occurred until the skin ulcerates over the undermined deep tissue.

PREVENTION

The key to prevention is the protection of vulnerable skin areas against pressure. The bedridden patient must be properly positioned to avoid pressure on bony prominences. When the patient is on his back, cushions should be placed under his legs to keep the heels from touching the bed sheet. In the lateral position, a pillow behind the back is adjusted in such a way that there is a minimum degree of pressure on the trochanter. The ankles may be wrapped in heavy protective dressings in order to avoid pressure on the malleoli. The skin must be kept clean, dry, and properly lubricated. The chief responsibility for proper skin care rests with the nurse, and technical details are presented in textbooks on nursing. Patients at risk must be turned every 2 hr during the day and at least every 4 hr at night. At no time should patients be permitted to lie on skin areas which show evidence of actual or impending breakdown. Preventive positioning and frequent turning are mandatory if patients are paralyzed or move very little on their own. The lethargic, poorly nourished, or incontinent patient particularly requires meticulous preventive skin care.

Patients with spinal cord lesions are especially vulnerable to the development of pressure sores over the anesthetic portions of their bodies. The routine of frequent turning must be established immediately after the injury. These patients should be turned from side to side in rotation. They should spend as little time as possible on their backs. They should sleep on their abdomen at night if possible since the pressure on bony prominences is minimal in the prone position. As early as possible, patient and family must be made aware of the dangers of skin breakdown. They must become active and knowledgeable partners in the preventive program. Most of these patients are young, and the risk of developing pressure sores will be with them for the rest of their lives. Before patients are discharged from the hospital they must have learned all aspects of skin care. They must inspect skin daily for areas of irritation and use a hand mirror to examine the lower back and buttocks. An area of persistent reddening, blanching, or blister formation must not be subjected to any pressure whatever until the irritation has subsided. This may entail time lost from school or job, but in the end this precautionary measure will pay off in the saving of time and spare the patient a costly period of prolonged hospitalization and surgical repair. It is often difficult to make paraplegic patients understand the hazards of skin breakdown since they feel no pain in the afflicted areas. We show our patients slides of pressure ulcers before they are discharged from the hospital in order to heighten their awareness.

In some hospitals paraplegic patients are placed on Stryker frames or circoelectric beds to prevent or heal ulcers. These devices are uncomfortable, and we have found that skin problems can be managed just as well in a hospital bed as long as the rules of proper positioning and turning are meticulously observed. The alternating air-pressure mattress consists of vertical air-filled chambers which run the length of the mattress and are about 3 inches wide. They are inflated and deflated by a motor in alternation. In this fashion no one skin area is exposed to pressure for any length of time. This mattress is a valuable adjunct to the prevention and care of decubitus ulcer, but it does not absolve the nurse from turning the patient frequently and from keeping the skin clean and dry. The use of this mattress must not create a false sense of security.

A large variety of cushions has been designed both for use in the wheelchair and in bed. As pointed out before, a 2-inch foam rubber cushion reduces the pressure on the ischial tuberosities to one-half.[1] More effective are flotation pads which are made from a viscoelastic gel encased in latex rubber. It protects the skin not only against pressure but also against lateral shearing forces. Its consistency is similar to human fat. The flotation pads offer good protection to vulnerable skin areas. They are heavy, however, and the latex rubber cover causes perspiration. In bed these pads are placed in a center cutout of a 2-inch foam rubber leveling mattress which is put on top of the ordinary mattress. The pad is positioned under the buttocks and lower back. Other cushions are filled with water, air, polyurethane foam impregnated with water, or latex foam. A newer type of cushion consists of 72 air-filled balloons; it is marketed under the name of Roho cushion. Most patients find this cushion comfortable. An additional advantage is that the weight distribution can be adjusted to need by tying the base of some of the balloons with rubber bands. DeLateur et al. studied the efficacy of seven cushions in paraplegic patients.[9] The cushions were used in rotation. The patient sat motionless on each cushion for 30 min. After the patient returned to bed, the duration of the reactive hyperemia was measured with a stop watch. Hyperemia was observed in all patients on any cushion. No significant differences between the seven cushion types were noted. The authors concluded that it is not possible to sit motionless on any of the cushions without some degree of hyperemia. It follows that paraplegic patients must be taught to shift their weight by push-ups many times within an hour in order to relieve skin surfaces from undue pressure.

THE TREATMENT OF DECUBITUS ULCERS

Decubitus ulcers are classified according to the degree of involvement.[10] A Grade I ulcer is limited to the epidermal and dermal layers. In these ulcers sebacious glands undergo necrosis, while hair follicles remain intact. A Grade II ulcer penetrates into subcutaneous fat layers. The adnexal structures from which reepithelialization may occur have been destroyed. A Grade III ulcer extends through all of the subcutaneous layers to muscle and into muscle. These ulcers are often extensively undermined. Grade IV ulcers show a destruction of all soft tissues and penetrate to the bone. The undermining is extensive.

Grade I ulcers can be managed conservatively. The key to treatment is to relieve the involved area of all pressure. If the epidermis and only the epidermis has undergone necrosis reepithelialization will occur. The deep adnexal cutaneous structures serve as foci for epithelial regeneration.

Grade II ulcers have a necrotic base in the subcutaneous tissue. The necrotic tissue must be removed before healing can take place. The wound is irrigated with hydrogen peroxide, then with saline and finally with betadine solution. This procedure must be carried out at least 3 times in 24 hr. An enzyme-containing ointment, Elase Ointment® (Parke-Davis), is useful in digesting and removing necrotic material. The active ingredients are fibrinolysin and desoxyribonuclease. The ulcer is covered with dry sterile dressings. No weight bearing is allowed. A Grade II ulcer will heal after several weeks or months. However, the skin may lack elasticity, and the epithelial layer is thin and inadequately keratinized, making it vulnerable to further injury.

Grade III and IV ulcers require surgical closure, but before this can be done, infections need to be cleared up and dead tissue must be removed. This requires frequent surgical debridement. The ulcer is packed with saline-soaked fine mesh gauze. Badly infected cavities are packed with iodoform gauze. A recent development has been the packing with a dextran polymer prepared in the form of dry porous beads.[11] This material absorbs fluid and protein-containing exudate and forms a protective gel cover. The material is quite expensive, and it has yet to be demonstrated that this treatment has advantages over gauze packing. The surgical repair usually consists of the removal of bony prominences and coverage with a skin flap. Obviously this should not be attempted until the base of the ulcer consists of clean, viable, and infection-free granulation tissue. It may take several weeks before the ulcer is ready for surgical closure. If the ulcer is deep, the cavity should be filled with muscle tissue, which forms the base of the flap. Postoperatively, adequate drainage is provided to prevent the accumulation of fluid or blood under the flap. The repaired area must be protected against pressure and tension for several weeks. This makes for a long postoperative period which the patient will have to spend in bed positioned on his abdomen.

The primary closure of ulcers is ineffective and is not recommended. Skin grafts are indicated only over non-weight-bearing areas since the grafted skin is delicate and breaks down easily.

Over the years, various methods of treating decubitus ulcers have been proposed. A few of these should be mentioned, even though none have found a wide acceptance. Ulcers have been packed with gelatin sponges,[12] sugar, or gold-leaf.[13] Hyperbaric oxygen has been used over ulcer cavities,[14] and low-intensity direct electrical currents were reported to stimulate the growth of granulation tissue.[15] None of these methods has stood the test of time. Furthermore, it is difficult to evaluate new therapeutic measures for pressure ulcers objectively and to establish valid controls. All therapeutic trials have a built-in placebo effect which must be taken into account. The heightened interest of the investigator will make him pay more than the usual attention to the patient's ulcerated skin. As a result patients on a therapeutic trial study will receive better than ordinary care.

This point has been well demonstrated by Fernie and Dornan.[16] These authors designed a machine equipped only with a number of switches and a cooling fan for the sound effect. The machine did nothing whatever but the nurses were told that it emitted an electromagnetic radiation from a metal cone and that the power of radiation could be varied by operating the different switches. Five patients with pressure ulcers that had been resistant to the usual methods of treatment were "treated" with this placebo device. The ulcers were exposed to the device day and night for 30 min out of every 2 hr. One ulcer healed completely within 14 days, and another healed 90 percent in 28 days. In the other three patients the size of the ulcer was decreased from 50 to 60 percent in a span of 14–20 days. Clearly, similar controlled studies will have to be devised to test the validity of treatment methods.

Of all organs the skin is most vulnerable to the noxious effects of immobilization. Pressure ulcers, however, can be prevented by good medical and nursing care. Once they occur they increase mortality, especially in elderly, chronically ill, and poorly nourished patients. In any case pressure ulcers contribute significantly to the morbidity, length of hospitalization, and cost of care. It has been estimated that a pressure sore increases the cost of care of a paraplegic patient by 150 percent.[6] Insurance companies are said to allot 25 percent of the estimated cost of care of a paraplegic patient for the treatment of decubitus ulcers.

REFERENCES

1. Kosiak, M., Kubicek, W. G., Olson, M., Danz, J. N., and Kottke, F. J. Evaluation of pressure as a factor in the production of ischial ulcers. *Arch. Phys. Med. Rehab.* **39**:623, 1958.

2. Bush, C. A. Study of pressures on the skin under ischial tuberosities and thighs during sitting. *Arch. Phys. Med. Rehab.* **50**:207, 1969.
3. Lindan, O. Etiology of decubitus ulcers: An experimental study. *Arch. Phys. Med. Rehab.* **42**:774, 1961.
4. Kosiak, M. Etiology and pathology of ischemic ulcers. *Arch. Phys. Med. Rehab.* **40**:62, 1959.
5. Reichel, S. M. Shearing force as a factor in decubitus ulcers in paraplegics. *J. Am. Med. Assoc.* **166**:762, 1958.
6. Dinsdale, S. M. Decubitus ulcers: Role of pressure and friction in causation. *Arch. Phys. Med. Rehab.* **55**:147, 1974.
7. Moolten, S. E. Bedsores in the chronically ill patient. *Arch. Phys. Med. Rehab.* **53**:430, 1972.
8. Exton-Smith, A. N. Prevention of pressure sores: monitoring mobility and assessment of clinical condition. In: *Bedsore Biomechanics* (R. M. Kenedi and J. M. Cowden, eds.), pp. 133–139. Baltimore, 1976. University Park Press.
9. DeLateur, B. J., Berni, R., Hongladarom, T., and Giaconi, R. Wheelchair cushions designed to prevent pressure sores: An evaluation. *Arch. Phys. Med. Rehab.* **57**:129, 1976.
10. Enis, J. E., and Sarmiento, A. The pathophysiology and management of pressure sores. *Orthop. Rev.* **2**:25, 1973.
11. Jacobsson, S., Rothman, U., Arturson, G., Ganrot, K., Haeger, K., and Juhlin, I. A new principle for the cleansing of infected wounds. *Scand. J. Plast. Reconstr. Surg.* **10**:65, 1976.
12. Young, C. G., and Oden, P. W. Treatment of decubitus ulcer in paraplegic patients. *South. Med. J.* **66**:1375, 1973.
13. Wolf, M., Wheeler, P. C., and Wolcott, L. E. Gold-leaf treatment of ischemic skin ulcers. *J. Am. Med. Assoc.* **196**:693, 1966.
14. Fischer, B. H. Topical hyperbaric oxygen treatment of pressure sores and skin ulcers. *Lancet* **2**:405, 1969.
15. Wolcott, L. E., Wheeler, P. C., Hardwicke, H. M., and Rowley, B. A. Accelerated healing of skin ulcers by electrotherapy. *South. Med. J.* **62**:795, 1969.
16. Fernie, G. R., and Dornan, J. The problems of clinical trials with new systems for preventing or healing decubiti. In: *Bedsore Biomechanics* (R. M. Kenedi, and J. M. Cowden, eds.), pp. 315–320. Baltimore, 1976. University Park Press.

CHAPTER 7

The Psychological Aspects of Immobilization

by
Randy L. Hammer, Ph.D.,
and
Emily H. Kenan, M.A.

INTRODUCTION

Until recent decades, the concept of immobilization, when thought of at all, conjured up visions of purely physical restraints such as body casts, restraining straps, or confinement to bed. Although certain obvious physical side effects of immobilization were recognized quite early in medical practice, they were generally regarded as unfortunate but sometimes necessary. And there the matter rested.

Attempts were made to relieve some of the discomforts, but little effort was expended to look further into the plight of the immobilized. During World War II, with its resulting casualties, the number of patients requiring immobilization increased, and this led to improved methods of treating the immobilized individual. However, even when forward-looking space scientists began considering the possible effects of prolonged space travel under confining conditions, the emphasis was more on the physical and physiological implications than on emotional and behavioral patterns. Still, a start was made and in the 1940s an examination of the psychological consequences of immobilization began.

The early approaches, understandably, tended to follow conventionally narrow concepts in which the immobilized patient was viewed as existing in a prisonerlike state, physically restrained by an external force or tediously confined to a bed. Such imagery was not without foundation. Asher[1] was among the first to describe some of the major hazards of bed rest in an effort to discourage physicians from prescribing this form of immobilization so readily. His attitude is summed up in the quote at the end of Chapter 1. In 1944 Phyllis Greenacre, writing one of the first papers to appear on the incidence and use of restrictive conditions or devices, associated forms of restraint with the then common practice of tying children's hands to discourage such activities as thumbsucking or masturbation.[2] Greenacre's paper also dealt with the less frequent instances in which a child might intentionally be kept in medical isolation for specific therapeutic management of infection or disease—and those even rarer episodes of children kept in "near-embalmed" or ambulatory catatonic states by disturbed or misguided parents.

With the benefits of hindsight, we may wonder how, with the clear recognition that confinement to bed and forms of restraints had negative, even fearful connotations, the rather obvious psychological and emotional implications of the matter so consistently escaped the notice of these early researchers. Yet, even today, the paucity of reported data on the subject of immobilization, particularly from a psychoanalytic point of view, indicates that this field of investigation may offer greater opportunities than has generally been supposed.

Before discussing the more recent attention given to the subject of immobilization, it may be helpful to know how the concept of immobilization, its various forms and manifestations, has expanded over the years. Therefore, precise definitions and classifications will be presented first.

IMMOBILIZATION DEFINED

Merriam-Webster defines *immobilize* as "to prevent the freedom of movement or effective use of; to reduce or eliminate motion (of the body or a part) by mechanical means or by strict bed rest."[3] This definition reflects the narrowness of the lay person's viewpoint traditionally associated with a subject not fully understood.

Spencer, Vallbona, and Carter similarly offer as the definition of immobilization, "the physical restriction or limitation of motion of body members and of the body in turning, sitting and ambulation."[4] They add, however, "This state may accompany extreme physical inactivity in critical illness where there is extensive motor paralysis and movement is not possible, or where there are restrictive physical postures, or as a result of therapy such as plaster casting, splinting, corseting, and binding. Physical restriction can be a consequence of physical environmental constraints like those imposed in a space capsule arrangement or when a person is confined within a full-body tank respirator." These authors are here broadening the picture to include such immobilizing factors as paralysis and one's physical environment—a step forward.

Becker also expanded the concept of restraint in that he included the ideas of restrictive cognitive and restrictive emotional environments, "where exposure to intrasensory or known stimulating experience may be systematically (though inadvertently or insensitively) denied over a long period . . . during periods of hospitalization."[5] Carnevali and Brueckner merely state that immobilization includes "the prescribed or unavoidable restriction of movement in any area of the patient's life."[6] This deceptively simple statement is important for its sensitivity to the fact that there are other aspects of immobilization which affect "any area of a patient's life"—by implication, the social, intellectual, and emotional limitations which are included, along with the physical restrictions placed on the patient.

In general, a review of these definitions indicates that the concept of immobilization has expanded as our knowledge and understanding have developed. In the simplest of terms, immobilization is the restriction of movement imposed directly to the body by a mechanical means. In broader terms, immobilization includes the limitation of physical activity caused by the individual's physical condition or by environmental confinement. The concept of immobilization can further be applied to an environment which is void of sensory stimulation. In addition, immobilization includes any area in an individual's life in which activities and interactions—intellectual, emotional, and social—are reduced.

The authors have taken the preceding definitions into account and have classified immobilization in two forms.

The first form is viewed as a restriction within the environment which prohibits or limits physical activity. This includes both restrictive measures applied directly to the body, such as braces, casts, and Stryker frames, as well as those imposed confinement to a restricted space (bed, intensive care unit, etc.). Thus, in this form, movement is physically possible but not allowed or restricted by external means.

The second form refers to restrictive factors relating to a

patient's physical or cognitive condition which inhibits movement or activity in any functional area of the patient's life. Such lack of movement is experienced by those in which movement is painful, the critically ill, and the paralyzed. The restriction may also refer to impaired activities and to the individual's intellectual and emotional instability or social insecurity. This second form of immobilization is apparent, whereas the physician's order or the body cast on a patient, imposing confinement, illustrates the first, or external, form of immobilization. With the second form of immobilization, movement is permitted but not possible because of factors within the individual.

A further distinction must be made here between primary and secondary immobilization as it may apply to the classification of either form of immobilization. This is simply to say that there are circumstances in which both external and internal forms of immobilization may be present, and it is important to differentiate between which is the dominant or primary form.

In some instances this may seem to be a question of which form of immobilization occurs first. The primary or source form of immobilization should not be confused with secondary forms or resultant effects. For example, an internally immobilized patient, such as the paralyzed individual, may also be confined to an intensive care unit. In this sense the confinement is an external form of immobilization in that it is imposed by an environmental source—the physician. On the other hand, the situation in which the patient is immobilized in a body cast may also contain a form of internal immobilization in that the emotional activities of that individual may be limited or suppressed. In the first example, internal immobilization is primary while in the second, external immobilization is primary.

IMMOBILIZATION RESEARCH

In their efforts to identify and categorize the effects of immobilization, researchers have attempted to study immobilization by dividing it into the separate but interacting components of physical inactivity, physical restriction, and loss of sensory and motor stimuli (sensory deprivation). Because each of these components simulate immobilization in different ways and to different degrees, they have served as a basis for investigations from which inferences can be made to better understand and, therefore, deal with the potential effects of immobilization.

Physical inactivity. Based on research in the field of immobilization, the component of physical inactivity has been shown to have negative effects on the total functioning of individuals in a variety of situations, whether the individual is disabled or not. One study designed to determine the physiologic and metabolic effects of physical inactivity, was conducted by Spencer, Vallbona, and Carter.[4] Subjects included a group of patients with various illnesses and injuries. In the case of one experimental subgroup, paralyzed individuals, the authors found that the effects of physical inactivity on the central nervous system lead to "decreased attention span; alterations in body image perception; behavioral regression; depression; emotional lability; alterations in visual motor coordination." Similarly, Riklan and Levita[7] and Plaski, Levita, and Riklan[8] studying the movement impairment of Parkinsonian patients, reported that the degree of inactivity or incapacitation was associated with reliable and pervasive intellectual and perceptual losses along with impoverishment of personality resources.

Oster points out that studies on astronauts demonstrate that inactivity results in a number of central nervous system changes such as electroencephalographic alterations, ineffectual behavior, and abnormalities in reflex time responses.[9]

Kottke,[10] who studied the impairment of emotional control and intellectual performance resulting from the prolonged inactivity of bed rest says,

> Bed rest which deprives the individual of intellectual stimulation has a progressively stultifying effect on intellectual activity.... Emotional response to diminution of activity will vary depending on the degree of sensory deprivation and the dominant personality factors of the individual. The immediate emotional response to limitation of activity is similar to that in other stress situations, and persons may show evidence of insecurity with anxiety and dependency or aggressiveness with hostility. Anxiety, hostility, tension, complaints of discomfort, and changes in sleep patterns all may occur in varying degrees depending upon the personality of the individual. The greater the degree and the more prolonged the limitation of activity and isolation, the greater will be the regression toward dependency and emotional responses.

It is obvious that Kottke has attributed a multitude of factors to be at work in producing the psychological deterioration. Although he speaks of physical inactivity as the primary cause of such deterioration, he closely associates sensory deprivation and the individual's premorbid personality with the impact of physical inactivity.

It is reasonable to hypothesize that many mental and behavioral changes or disturbances may be due to physical inactivity which limits environmental, intellectual, and social input as well as sensory–kinesthetic feedback derived from movement itself.

Physical restriction. A second component of immobilization, physical restriction, is conceptualized as a form of immobilization in which an external source is preventing activity.

Freedman, Grunebaum, and Greenblatt[11] note that the effects of restricted voluntary movement upon humans have not been separately and sufficiently subjected to carefully controlled experimentation. They voice their suspicion that critical differences in individuals' functioning may be due to the degree of movement permitted. After reviewing a number of studies, they state that "in every instance of restricted motility, hallucinations have been reported, while in two experimental situations with free motility, minimal or no hallucinations were reported."

A series of Canadian experiments[12-14] has shown that subjects whose physical activity or level of kinesthetic-proprioceptive stimulation was reduced for a week by external immobilization (physical restriction), but who otherwise were not deprived of sensory input, exhibited a variety of cognitive and perceptual motor deficits. These defects included unusual subjective phenomena and a slowing of the electrical activity of the brain.

Such data clearly illustrate the impact of restricted movement in terms of psychological effects upon the individual's abilities. However, even stronger evidence exists in the investigations of the relationship between the onset of surgical casting in connection with a wide range of orthopedic procedures, with subsequent immobilization of the child-patient and the inhibition of verbal expression. Other researchers[15-17] observed that if the casting occurred at an age that might be concurrent with the development of speech and language (ages 18 months to 3 years), children would regress in verbalization, or, when just having learned to speak, would lose that behavioral expression altogether.

Levy's study on the psychological outcomes of early motor restriction noted that when children are "liberated" from their confinement, they often showed a tendency to be disorderly and hyperkinetic for some time afterward.[15] These children became behaviorally unmanageable and found it quite difficult to maintain their attentiveness for any prolonged period of time in connection with their school work. They also exhibited thought pressure, rapid or racing ideational output, or other intersensory evidence of integrative disinhibition of function.

Sensory deprivation. The majority of experimental work has been conducted on a third component of immobilization, sensory deprivation or sensory isolation. The result of Zubek's studies[12-14] demonstrate that increasing the extent of the immobilized condition by the additional deprivation of visual and auditory stimulation, produces even greater behavioral impairments than does physical inactivity or physical restriction alone. This was shown particularly by a significant deficit in depth perception and size constancy.[18]

In an experiment conducted by Heron, subjects were required to lie in bed in a lighted cubicle 24 hr a day for as long as they would stay.[19] Visual, auditory, and tactile input were severely restricted, and a wide variety of behaviors was measured. Gross disturbances occurred in cognitive, perceptual, and motor performance as a result of this sensory deprivation. The subjects reported that their thought processes gradually underwent changes, eventually reaching the point where visual, auditory, and somatic hallucinations occurred. Several subjects reported peculiar sensations of touch and movement, such as electric shocks, experiencing the presence of another body lying beside or overlapping their own, and general "bodily strangeness." In addition, the experimenters noted that the subjects became quite irritable, childish, and suspicious toward them.

Edith J. Olson points out that a number of "clinical studies indicate that sensory deprivation causes a decrease in the perceptions of pattern and form, weight discrimination, pressure, and temperature sensitivity. It also tends to decrease the speed of perception."[20] Another major finding from Olson's work points out the varied distortion of time. More specifically, this entails an inaccuracy of time estimation and a confusion of past, present, and future sequencing.

Looking more closely into sensory deprivation, Lilly attempted to answer the question of what happens to a brain in the relative absence of physical stimuli.[21] In preparing to do this, Lilly explored pertinent autobiographical literature concerned with accounts by persons who were survivors of social isolation, either in the polar regions or at sea. The most obvious overall finding is that isolation per se acts on most persons as a powerful stress. Other findings characteristic among the survivors included: delusions (of the "savior" type rather than a "destroyer" type), reliance on superstitions, intense love of any living things, conversations with inanimate objects, a new inner security and new integration of themselves on a deep and basic level, with a feeling that when rescued, one had best be careful to listen before speaking to avoid being considered insane.

Although the underlying mechanisms accounting for these disturbances remain obscure, these experiences clearly indicate that certain inner mental factors tend to be projected outward—"that some of the mind's activity which is usually reality-bound now becomes free to turn to fantasy and, ultimately, to hallucination and delusion."[21]

Lilly's literature review led to a study in which the method was to reduce the absolute intensity of all physical stimuli to the lowest point.[21] Two subjects with a maximum exposure of 3 hr were involved. The subjects were immersed in a tank of slowly flowing water at 34.5°C (94.5°F) approximating normal body temperature, so that sensations of hot or cold were not felt. The head, which remained above water, was completely covered with a blackout mask. Subjects were later asked to write notes on their experiences and sensations, which are sequentially summarized as follows:

1. For about the first 45 min, residues of the day's sensory experiences continued to be predominant.
2. Gradually, a sense of relaxation, even enjoyment, developed.
3. During the following hour a tension or "stimulus-action" hunger was noted; hidden methods of self-stimulation occurred.
4. As the "hunger" grew, the whole content of consciousness focused on any available residual stimulation to an almost unbearable degree.
5. At the next stage, thoughts shifted from direct thinking about problems to highly personal, emotionally charged reveries and fantasies.
6. Finally, projections of visual imagery were experienced.

The longest experimentally controlled exposure to isolation, involving the largest number of subjects, was carried out by Donald Hebb and a group of graduate students at McGill University.[22] Similar to Lilly's research,[21] the aim was to reduce stimuli to the lowest level and to observe and record the results. To accomplish this, subjects in the McGill University study were placed in a bed in an air-conditioned box with arms and hands restrained with cardboard sleeves. Their eyes were covered completely with translucent ski goggles. The subjects, college students motivated by payment of $20 per day for as long as they would stay in the box, were observed through a window and tested verbally via a communication set. Although the subjects' details of their experiences varied considerably, a few general phenomena appeared.

> After several hours, each subject found that it was diffi-
> cult to carry on organized, directed thinking for any sus-
> tained period. Suggestibility was very much increased.
> An extreme desire for stimuli and action developed. There
> were periods of thrashing around in the box in attempts
> to satisfy this need. The borderline between sleep and
> awakedness became diffuse and confused. At some time
> between 24 to 72 hours most subjects could not stand it
> any longer and left. Hallucinations and delusions of
> various sorts developed, mostly in those who could stay
> longer than two days.

The results of such laboratory research on sensory isolation parrallel those found in cases of polar and sea isolation,
of which it is said, "If one is alone long enough, and at levels
of physical and human stimulation low enough, the mind
turns inward and projects outward its own contents and
processes; the brain not only stays active despite the lowered
levels of input and output, but accumulates surplus energy
to extreme degrees."[21]

Zubek, Heron, Olson, Lilly, and Heron[18–22] all indicate
that in the absence of stimuli, the cognitive processes
undergo a number of changes. With minimal to moderate
degrees of sensory isolation, thoughts become less organized
and less directed. In cases of more extreme and lengthy isolation, the cognitive processes shift from reality-bound activities to fantasy, and finally to hallucinations. In addition, certain similar aftereffects of isolation have been noted. At the
conclusion of research conducted by the Hebb group, subjects had difficulty in orienting their perceptual mechanisms
and various illusions persisted for hours. The Lilly subjects
felt "out of step" with the clock for the rest of the day, and
reported the need to readjust to social intercourse in a variety

of ways. Similarly, the survivors of polar and sea isolation needed time before socially interacting, in which to reestablish a sense of reality or "saneness."

The previous research has been of laboratory-controlled experiments in which the individuals were deprived of sensory input far greater than found in most real-life situations. Rarely do we find an individual who is restricted from all the sources of stimuli at the same time and to such a degree. However, in the case of the immobilized individual there are extensive reductions of sensory input, although not to the same extent.

We know that immobilization means a reduction of physical activity. We also know that this physical inactivity is apt to result in the individual being confined to a specific area. The confinement may result in a degree of environmental sameness and a decrease in sensory stimuli. The confinement may also result in fewer opportunities for social interaction—a source of sensory stimulation that has been given little attention so far.

One of the major sources of environmental stimulation found in man's everyday life is received from interacting with others. Not only are auditory, olfactory, and visual stimulation involved, but intellectual and emotional stimulation as well. Social interaction is not commonly thought of as necessary for life. It has been shown that infants deprived of physical contact, however, do not live. Thus, the need for human interaction is essential in the early stages of human existence. As the child develops, the need for interaction may change in nature but not in significance. Interaction with human beings enables the child to establish a sense of self-reality as separate from, but part of, a real world. Continued interaction maintains a sense of direction and a feeling of belonging.

It is no small wonder that in the experiences of social isolation, either in polar regions or at sea, the survivors found themselves placing high value on conversing with inanimate objects. In some cases individuals were completely devoid of human contact. In others, where there were two or more survivors, the available human contact was not sufficient. Only the objects within the environment, outside of the personal experience, could serve as a basis of reality. The survivors needed to relate to these objects for the necessary stimulation and reality orientation to remain alive. Unfortunately, however, specific information comparing the experience of the survivors who were deprived of all human contact with those who were not is unavailable. Similarly, in much of the sensory deprivation research all of the subjects were deprived of human interaction; thus the effects of social isolation were not separately subject to controlled experimentation.[18-20,22]

IMMOBILIZATION APPLIED

Having demonstrated that the three components of immobilization—physical inactivity, physical restriction, and sensory deprivation (which includes social isolation)—prove detrimental to a person's functional abilities, we must now look at the interaction of these components. The information provided gives rise to the supposition that these components involve a cyclical and cumulative process of deterioration.

As discussed previously, immobilization causes a number of physical, intellectual, emotional, and social changes which disturb the individual's life. Each of these disturbances, in turn, causes more changes, leading to more intensified disturbances. These changes and disturbances represent a cyclical pattern, which increasingly affects the individual's overall stability. Another way of describing this same process is that immobilization, external or internal, leads to self-perpetuating, secondary forms of immobilization. This becomes clearer if immobilization is thought of in terms of how it is experienced by the individual.

The most obvious aspect of immobilization is a reduction of physical activity. It may be due to an external restriction imposed by the environment which directly limits or prohibits freedom of physical movement. Or, the immobilization may be due to internal restrictive factors relating to a patient's physical or cognitive condition which inhibits movement or activity in any functional area of the patient's life. In this case, movement is permitted, physically and environmentally, but is not possible for other reasons.

Whether immobility is externally or internally imposed, a degree of confinement will result. Remaining confined will decrease the sensory stimulation (intellectually, emotionally, socially, physically, and environmentally) due to limited movement, environmental constancy, and fewer social interactions. The lack of stimulation can lead to a dulling of the individual's sensory receptivity since individuals maintain contact with the environment through the senses by responding to the perceived sensory stimuli. When there is a reduction in the quantity and quality of sensory stimulation available to the organism, the efficiency of the sensory processing system decreases. The individual does not respond effectively—intellectually, emotionally, physically, or socially. As a result, the individual experiences the cumulative effects of further immobilization of an internal nature. In other words, the immobilization factors from that point on are internally or self-imposed rather than externally or environmentally imposed. Thus, the immobilization cycle may be visualized as below:

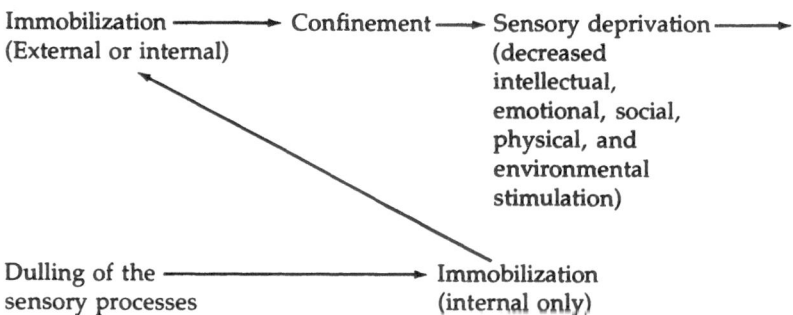

Immobilization ⟶ Confinement ⟶ Sensory deprivation ⟶
(External or internal)   (decreased
                                        intellectual,
                                        emotional, social,
                                        physical, and
                                        environmental
                                        stimulation)

Dulling of the ⟶ Immobilization
sensory processes   (internal only)

A summary of the findings related to the intellectual, emotional and social effects of immobilization will be helpful in understanding how this cyclical and cumulative process affects an individual.

Intellectual Effects. In the research on learning and motivation, studies of immobilized or isolated individuals have demonstrated subjects' decreased motivation to learn, retain, transfer, and generalize information. "In the area of problem-solving there were also lessened motivation, losses in ability to receive necessary content for problem-solving because of decreased sensory stimulation, and a decrease in the ability to discriminate."[20]

Kottke found that progressive dulling of the intellect gives way to confusion.[23] This confusion gives way to disinterest in eating, loss of attention to bladder and bowel condition, and a loss of interest in further activity. Progressively, loss of interest in or motivation for an activity may lead to less of that activity. This produces more difficulty or discomfort when eventually taking action—and this difficulty or discomfort inhibits the desire for more of the activity.

We can understand from this information that the person whose intellectual, emotional, physical, or social activities have been limited may be less inclined to initiate activity even when movement is permitted. The process becomes fully circular, self-intensifying, and self-destructive.

Emotional Effects

> Emotions are internal events of the organism demonstrated by bodily changes and by behavioral changes. Studies have indicated that drives and expectancies were greatly diminished by immobility, while emotions were expressed in various ways. Examples of emotional expression included apathy, withdrawal, frustrated anger, aggression or regression.[20]

Any form of change in an individual's patterns usually is accompanied by an emotional reaction, more intense than normal expressions. Sudden immobility, whether traumatic or therapeutic, will also set the stage for the expression of exaggerated or inappropriate emotional reactions. Common expressions are loss of personal worth, fear, wounded pride, guilt, disgust, anger, and frustration. In infants and young children, frustration is particularly obvious.[24] Since children theoretically function at more primitive levels than adults, with less defensiveness, they tend to express their emotions more openly when there is physical interference with their spontaneous motor activity.

At higher levels of psychological functioning, adults will more readily feel the emotional effects of immobilization in a more narcissistic way—in terms of their body image for example. The intimate association of body image with one's sense of personal worth and of one's proper place among other people goes even deeper. Numerous studies point out that an individual's conception of his or her body as a whole or of different body parts, greatly contributes to the personality, affect, and interpersonal relationships. The immobilized individual will very likely have to contend with such bodily changes as weight loss, atrophy, decreased bulk, and new postural images (i.e., sitting in a wheelchair or ambulating with various orthoses). Whereas such changes are the source of much discomfort for adults, several analysts investigating body image disturbances in children state that they introject and incorporate the objects of their (external) immobilization, such as braces, prosthetic devices, etc., into their body-image concepts.[5]

In assessing the effects of immobilization on adults, one must take into account the cultural determinants in this country. Americans place much emphasis on youth, vigor, strength, physique, wholeness, and constant activity. In a society which stresses such features, the disabled and consequently immobilized adult feels diminished in his/her personal worth. It must also be remembered that immobilized patients have the additional stress of fear—fear of the new alien environment, fear of death or mutilation, fear of abandonment and, most importantly, fear of rejection. The response to these fears can be depression and anxiety with associated agitation.

Hyman states, "Loss of mobility leads to loss of independence, both financial and personal. Coupled with loss of the patient's home, loss of loved ones, and establishment of a poor self-image, the result is a pronounced deprivation of previous values."[25] Much of this loss and/or deprivation leads to a pronounced regression of emotions as well as behavior. Unfortunately, while the patient is having to deal with emotional issues in a regressive manner, he or she is often hospitalized. The hospital milieu, particularly for a newly disabled/immobilized individual, can be viewed as one in which regressive tendencies are fostered, since all basic needs (feeding, clothing, shelter, and even bowel and bladder care in many instances) are taken care of for the patient.

The loss of independent status or self-esteem even for a short period of time, tends to be reflected in the patient's emotional status, primarily in the form of regressive, egocentric demands. In addition, these changes in the patient's emotions and behaviors can alter the patient's social habits as well.

Social Effects. An individual feeling any of the above described emotions may feel less inclined, if at all, to interact socially. At the same time, others may find social interaction with individuals displaying those emotions and behaviors undesirable.

In addition to changes in social interactions, social roles change through decreased physical activity, decreased occupational activity, and decreased sensory and motor interaction for social responsibility and cultural participation. Again, there are social forces at work. In a society which places prime value on the worker role, the nonworker role is generally to be interpreted as a movement to a lesser position, with consequent lowering of status in the social hierarchy. Furthermore, "the roles of spouse, parent, sexual partner, employee, club member, and leader may be altered, reversed or eliminated."[20] The disturbances in drives, expectations, emotions, intellect, roles, and values make social interactions more difficult. The patient withdraws. Social isolation lowers the individual's sensitivity to social cues and thus makes it more difficult to have the attitudinal and behavioral prerequisites to successful interactions and relationships.

A number of studies indicate that social isolation is indeed a significant factor to be considered. Martin D. Hyman found that loneliness, lack of social integration, and living alone are all somewhat detrimental to a patient's performance (motivation and functional improvement) in rehabilitation settings.[25] Hyman summarized the results of preceding studies:

> Litman[26] found that orthopedically disabled patients who had engaged in little social participation prior to treatment displayed substantially less motivation in a program of physical rehabilitation than did the more socially active patients. Sussman[27] reports that tuberculosis patients who did not live with a family member were significantly less likely, following treatment, to have achieved adequate medical, vocational, economic, and social rehabilitation. Bolton et al.[28] found that having dependents was conducive to successful vocational rehabilitation. Roth and Eddy[29] describe the manner in which lack of social contact raises the odds against a successful outcome for patients with a variety of ailments in the rehabilitation ward of a large public hospital.[25]

An increasing amount of evidence, derived from studies of a variety of populations and treatment programs, demonstrates that the degree of social isolation (prior to, during, and after treatment) cannot only impair rehabilitation but can adversely affect the seeking of treatment. Conversely, such evidence indicates the importance for the patient to be in close contact with a significant other. In some cases staff may act as surrogate friends and relatives. As Litman points out, the patient needs a sense of social support and encouragement in order to enhance the patient's motivation which, in turn, contributes markedly to the ability to respond to treatment.[26] Roth and Eddy also emphasize the importance of the patient having an advocate.[29] Their findings reveal that the patients who had someone guiding and protecting them, making sure the needed care was received, responded more rapidly and effectively to treatment.

Countering the Effects of Immobilization. Since the mere fact of illness and therapy is bound to change the patient's normal life patterns, it can be said that practically all patients will experience some of the psychological effects of immobilization. For these reasons, a specific treatment plan to meet the individual needs of each patient should be established so as to minimize sensory and social deprivation and maximize physical and mental functioning. Treatment programs should include medical and psychiatric management, physical, psychosocial, occupational, recreational, and speech therapies, as well as environment manipulation.

Psychological treatment consists of brief psychotherapy to prevent or curtail emotions or behaviors which may be harmful to the immobilized patient's overall stability. Psychotherapy can counter unnecessary regression, increase thoughts of independence, encourage problem solving, and permit emotional catharsis. It is most important that the patients not be allowed to sink into a state of emotional paralysis or lethargy. Neither should it be assumed that the patients can discuss their inner thoughts and feelings with a family member or a significant other. The therapist is made available as the one person to whom the patient can turn for objective understanding and guidance. The therapist helps the patient to verbalize any fears, doubts, conflicts, and needs, and to realize, accept, and adjust to changes in areas of his or her life.

Having the patient participate in group psychotherapy sessions is also recommended, in that it allows him or her to know that others are dealing with similar psychological and emotional difficulties and that peer "advocates" are available. In addition, the patients can learn from one another how to express themselves and how others have coped. Qualified individuals should also be available to aid significant others in healthy adjustment to patient changes. Another method of accomplishing this would be to encourage family members or "advocates" to participate in the patient's daily care and education. This participation should be undertaken with the ultimate goal of establishing appropriate amounts of future care without fostering an inordinate amount of regression or dependency.

Another helpful suggestion is to have a qualified individual, whether a psychologist, physician, or nurse, prepare the patient and significant others beforehand with information about what to expect from the hospitalization, thus decreasing stress and fear of the unknown, which can be felt as a loss of control, and subsequently lead to withdrawal (internal immobilization).

The importance of other hospital department participation is also warranted. Occupational therapy aids in reality orientation in that its goals are to increase the patient's ability to interact with the environment, thereby improving psychomotor functions for activities of daily living and identifying related areas that require realistic adaptations. In doing so, the therapy stimulates the emotional, intellectual, and social sensitivities of the patient. The patient is made to face the ways in which his or her life has changed and is thus helped to find and use alternatives that are consistent with his or her physical and mental abilities. Patients must work toward a degree of emotional acceptance and challenge their cognitive and physical processes to derive ways to best help themselves to return to their previous environment as independently or as "normally" as possible. Working toward or arriving at such an accomplishment also enhances self-esteem.

Barker, Wright, and Gonick point out that when a person is ill, the individual's world is reduced to his or her present condition and related concerns.[30] Occupational therapy is most helpful in aiding the patient to expand his or her thoughts beyond the present day to outside the hospital setting. The authors would like to point out that the presence of a television, a radio, newspapers, magazines, a clock, and a calendar in the patient's room will serve to help expand the patient's intellectual and emotional awareness. Also, if a patient's education has been interrupted by immobilization, the possibility of a tutor should be strongly considered to reinforce the patient's link to the "outside world."

Physicians have found that negative effects result if physical inactivity occurs for any length of time. Therefore, it is most important that the patient be prompted to move body parts as soon as their physical condition permits. Physical therapy offers a systematic and safe approach to facilitate proprioceptive input and thus inhibit physical deterioration as well as intellectual dulling.

Physical therapy may also improve self-concept/body-image concerns by allowing the patient to work with his physical appearance and physical abilities, thus giving him a sense of control over what is happening to his body. Working with one's body, looking at the changes in a mirror, and not hiding those changes from others, all help the individual to become more familiar with physical differences and therefore more accepting of them. Another way to improve self-concept is to have the patient dress in street clothes, when and where practical, which helps to dispel the "sick role" associated with a hospital gown. Buying new clothes, applying makeup, and having one's hair cut or styled should be supported because such actions indicate a positive interest in one's physical appearance. This is one way in which patients show their readiness to interact with others. Higher-level desired interactions with others may later take form in the patient's curiosity about sexual functioning.

Before the patients can feel comfortable with others, they must feel comfortable with themselves. Therefore, psychotherapy, physical therapy, speech therapy, and occupational therapy indirectly enhance comfortable interaction. These therapies are also conducive to social interaction in that they require the patient to interact with the therapist as well as with others who are present. Recreational therapy may go one step further by requiring the patient to actually go out into society. Placed in a social situation, social interactions do occur even if there are no verbal exchanges. Recreational therapy can allow the patient to "test the water."

Let us turn our attention to the patient who is not involved with any form of therapy at the moment. A variety of stimulation can be provided to that individual who is quietly sitting or lying in bed. The physical environment may be altered to be stimulating to the senses with decoration of the rooms to provide color, pleasing textures, comfortable levels of illumination, plants, fixtures, and familiar objects such as photos or mementos. The importance of newspapers, magazines, clocks, and calendars has already been mentioned.

Auditory stimulation is provided through television, radio, and record or tape player. The social environment is broadened by bedside visits, an accessible phone, and the availability of volunteer group activities involving the patient. Again, the importance of the patient's feeling that he or she has an advocate is stressed, since research has proven that the presence of an advocate positively influences the patient's social inclinations.[25,29]

In summary, most areas, of the patient's life are going to be affected by any of the various forms of immobilization. Immobilization does not merely refer to a form of limited activity; it also involves the consequences of that limitation— all of the resultant behavioral, intellectual, emotional, physical, and social changes experienced by the patient.

The information derived from research indicates that the major early warning signs of the negative effects of immobilization may be withdrawal, lack of energy, regression, decreased mental capacity, or in general, inappropriate or exaggerated responses. Patient exposure to as much varied stimulation as possible, from or with the help of as many people as possible, will most effectively counter or at least mitigate such occurrences. Efforts to understand that there are negative psychological and emotional implications related to immobilization, as well as efforts to take preventive measures, are the responsibility of all allied health professionals and of family members or significant others.

REFERENCES

1. Asher, R. A. J. The dangers of going to bed. *Br. Med. J.* **2**:967, 1947.
2. Greenacre, P. Infant reactions to restraint: Problems in the fate of infantile aggression. *Am. J. Orthopsychiatry* **14**:204, 1944.
3. Merriam-Webster. *Webster's New Collegiate Dictionary.* Springfield, Massachusetts, 1967. G. & C. Merriam Co.
4. Spencer, W. A., Vallbona, C., and Carter, R. E. Physiologic concepts of immobilization. *Arch. Phys. Med. Rehab.* **46**:1, 1965.
5. Becker, R. D. Recent developments in child psychiatry—clinical paediatrics liaison consultation. I. The restrictive emotional and cognitive environment reconsidered—a redefinition of the concept of therapeutic restraint. *Isr. Ann. Psychiatry Relat. Discip.* **13**:239, 1975.
6. Carnevali, D., and Brueckner, S. Immobilization. *Am. J. Nurs.* **70**:1502, 1970.
7. Riklan, M., and Levita, E. Psychological studies in Parkinsonism. Effects of subcortical surgery. *J. Gerontol.* **21**:372, 1966.
8. Ploski, H., Levita, E., and Riklan, M. Impairment of voluntary movement in Parkinson's Disease in relation to the activation level, autonomic malfunction, and personality rigidity. *Psychosom. Med.* **28**:70, 1966.
9. Oster, C. Sensory deprivation in geriatric patients. *J. Am. Geriatr. Soc.* **24**:461, 1976.

10. Kottke, F. J. The effects of limitation of activity upon the human body. *J. Am. Med. Assoc.* **196**:825, 1966

11. Freedman, S., Grunebaum, H., and Greenblatt, M. Perceptual and cognitive changes in sensory deprivation. In: *Sensory Deprivation* (Philip Solomon *et al.*, eds.). Cambridge, Massachusetts, 1961. Harvard University Press.

12. Zubek, J. P. Urinary excretion of adrenaline and noradrenaline during prolonged immobilization. *J. Abnorm. Psychol.* **73**:223, 1968.

13. Zubek, J. P., and MacNeill, M. Effects of immobilization: Behavioral and EEG changes. *Can. J. Psychol.* **20**:316, 1966.

14. Zubek, J. P., and Wilgosh, L. Prolonged immobilization of the body: Changes in performance and in the electroencephalogram. *Science* **140**:306, 1963.

15. Levy, D. M. On the problem of movement restraint; tics, stereo-typed movements, hyperactivity. *Am. J. Orthopsychiatry* **14**:644, 1944.

16. Bergmann, T. Observation of children's reactions to motor restraints. *Nerv. Child* **4**:318, 1945.

17. Burlingham, D. Notes on problems of motor restraint during illness. In: *Drives, Affects, Behavior* (R. M. Lowenstein, ed.), pp. 169–175. New York, 1953. International Universities Press.

18. Zubek, J. P.. Boyer, L., Milstein, S., and Shephard, J. M. Behavioral and physiological changes during prolonged immobilization plus perceptual deprivation. *J. Abnorm. Psychol.* **74**:230, 1969.

19. Heron, W. The pathology of boredom. In: *Frontiers of Psychosocial Research* (D. Coppersmith, ed.). San Francisco California, 1966. Freeman Press.

20. Olson, E. V. Effects of psychosocial equilibrium. *Am. J. Nurs.* **67**:794, 1967.

21. Lilly, J. C. Mental effects of physical restraint and of reduction of ordinary levels of physical stimuli on intact, healthy persons. *Psychiatr. Res. Rep.* **5**:1, 1956.

22. Heron, W., Bexton, W. H., and Hebb, D. O. Cognitive effects of a decreased variation to the sensory environment. *Am. Psychol.* **8**:366, 1953.

23. Kottke, F. J. Deterioration of the bedfast patient. *Public Health Rep.* **80**:437, 1965.

24. Vernon, D. T. A., Foley, J. M., Sipowicwz, R. R., and Schulman, J. L. *Psychological Responses of Children to Hospitalization and Illness.* Springfield, Illinois, 1965. Charles C Thomas.

25. Hyman, M. D. Social isolation and performance in rehabilitation. *J. Chronic Dis.* **25**:85, 1972.

26. Litman, T. J. *The Influence of Concept of Self and Life Orientation Factors*

upon the Rehabilitation of Orthopedic Patients. Ph.D. Dissertation, University of Minnesota, 1961.
27. Sussman, M. B. *Rehabilitation and Tuberculosis.* Cleveland, Ohio, 1964. Western Reserve University.
28. Bolton, B. F., Butler, A. J., and Wright, G. N. *Clinical versus Statistical Prediction of Client Feasibility.* Madison, 1968. The University of Wisconsin Regional Rehabilitation Research Institute.
29. Roth, A., and Eddy, E. M. *Rehabilitation for the Unwanted.* New York, 1967. Atherton Press.
30. Barker, R., Wright, B., and Gonick, M. *Adjustment to Physical Handicap and Illness: A Survey of the Social Psychology of Physique and Disability.* New York, 1946. Social Science Research Council.

Index

151